THE
DOG SAFETY
BIBLE

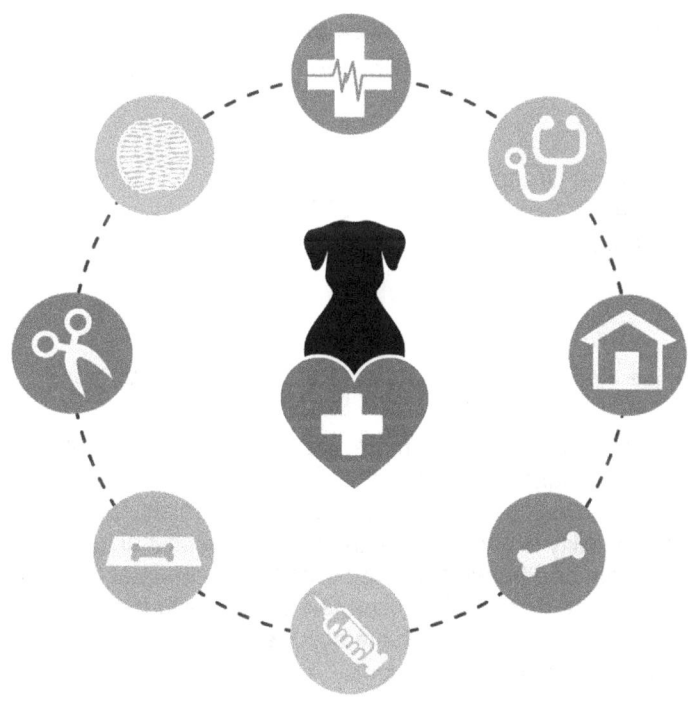

Dog Safety and First Aid For Your Dog

Denise Fleck and Robert Semrow

Pet World Media Group

Important Note Regarding Dog Care,
First-Aid & CPCR Techniques Provided In This Book

If you have any questions about your dog's health,
seek professional Veterinary care immediately!

These recommendations and the contents of this book are designed
to help you keep your dog more comfortable and aid with minor problems before
you are able to get to (or are on your way to) an animal hospital or Veterinarian's office.

They are not meant to be a substitute for care by a licensed Veterinary professional.

No liability is assumed by the authors, publisher or any other party with respect
to the information, suggestions and techniques described in this book.

Should there be any discrepancy between the suggestions offered
and the advice of a Veterinarian, it is recommended that the advice
of the Veterinarian be followed since the Veterinarian has the advantage
of physically examining the pet and knowing its medical history and circumstances.

Published by Pet World Media Group
4533 Mac Arthur Blvd. #340, Newport Beach, CA 92660
E-Mail: Info@petworldmediagroup.com
Phone: 888-969-7297

ISBN: 978-1-949695-04-5

First Edition

Printed and Manufactured in the United States of America

Information and updates on this book and other Pet World Media Group projects
can be found on www.petworldmediagroup.com

B&W Course Workbook Edition

TABLE OF CONTENTS

Section Two: Why You Should Know Canine First-Aid & CPCR

Dog First-Aid Conclusion

About the Authors

Section Three: Resources

Important Note Regarding Dog Care,
First-Aid & CPCR Techniques Provided In This Book

BEFORE YOU ADOPT

Sharing your life with a dog may be one of the most rewarding things you ever do during your lifetime…it totally ROCKS, but…it is a HUGE responsibility! Another living being will depend on you for its entire life, and YOU must make that life as safe and satisfying as possible. No matter what curves life throws your way, how much you change, get busy or tired, even if your income declines, you must keep your heart, schedule and home open for the dog you have made part of your family for its lifetime!

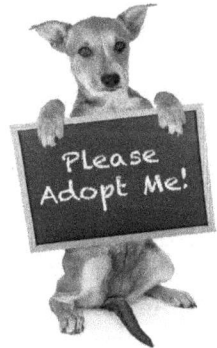

Caring for a four-legged friend takes time, money and energy, so you must be committed, willing to work hard and even make a compromise along the way to be a good dog parent.

CHOOSING YOUR DOG

Canis lupus familiaris (aka "man's and woman's best friend") is a domesticated subspecies of the Grey Wolf. Taming occurred nearly 15,000 years ago and the dog quickly became omnipresent in cultures across the globe. Dogs were extremely valuable to early human settlements, and in fact, it is often suggested that successful emigration across the Bering Strait may not have been possible without the help of dogs that pulled sleds of people and supplies. Currently, it is estimated that there are more than 400 million dogs in the world. Each breed and individual dog's abilities however are shaped by various genetic traits and learned behaviors. Some traits were intentionally bred by humans, while others were a result of the need to survive. Due to his wide range of traits, the dog has developed into hundreds of breeds representing more behavioral and physical variations than any other land mammal. The American Kennel Club (AKC) recognizes close to 200 different dog breeds not to mention the designer mixes that can be found most everywhere.

Dogs have a large variety of standardized and specialized needs. For instance, if you don't comb out your dog, he could get matted which can lead to uncomfortable sores and ultimately cause him to have to be shaved down at the groomers.

Puppies need house-breaking and training. Will you gladly get up every two hours during the night for feedings and bathroom breaks? Can you sleep through the incessant cries coming from the tiny furry creature who wants nothing more than to be cuddled by you at 3am? And maybe those cries shouldn't be ignored, so will you get up and see what is ailing your tiny pooch? How about those wet spots on the carpet (or the middle of your bed) until Rover learns that the great outdoors is his bathroom?

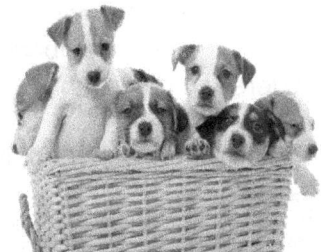

Puppies don't know the rules and require a patient human to teach them. When you adopt a small furry friend you must be prepared for sleepless nights, rushing home to let them out to answer nature's call and remain equipped with lots and lots of endless love.

Senior pets have it down...they know their manners, are calmer and even more focused. They are often perfectly content to let you go about your day lying by your side, thrilled for a pat on the head or the occasional belly rub. They just want to be with you, but as time goes by, they may require medical care. Is your bank account prepared for that? Patience again becomes of prime importance as accidents happen when pets get older. You will need to develop ways to make clean-up easier so that you never lose your temper with your best buddy. Ideas are discussed later in this book.

Large dogs need more space. It is definitely cramped with a Great Dane in a studio apartment, however...do your research regarding the breed and don't go on assumptions alone. A smaller Beagle or Basset Hound, who bays and howls or a yappy Chihuahua will not make your next door apartment neighbor happy either. Size isn't the only issue to consider. Also think about what sounds your dog might make and how loud he is in your absence.

Energetic breeds (hounds, shepherds, collies, spaniels, pointers, terriers and retrievers to name a few) require a securely fenced yard high enough that they can't jump it, but they also need to go on walks/runs, have the ball thrown and really expend that energy with you, their favorite person, several times a day. Do your research...

The nearly 200 breeds recognized by the American Kennel Club (AKC) have been separated into Sporting, Non-Sporting, Working, Hound, Terrier, Herding, Toy and Miscellaneous groups. However, there are other terms used to describe dogs that enlighten us to their abilities and needs. A dog can fall into several of these types, so knowing your dog's type can better help you know your dog.

Ancient or primitive dogs show the fewest genetic differences from the wolf and therefore most closely resemble their "canine cousins" in looks, temperament and drive. Breeds considered primitive include the Afghan, Akita, Alaskan Malamute, Chow Chow, Lhasa Apso, Basenji, Canaan Dog, Ibizan, New Guinea Singing Dog, Pekingese, Pharaoh Hound, Saluki, Shiba Inu, Samoyed, Siberian Husky and the Tibetan Terrier.

Barrel-chested dogs have round chests that provide these animals with maximum structural strength that resists compression. Students of Pet First-Aid know that sometimes CPCR is performed in a different fashion on these breeds since it's harder to compress their strong ribcage. Rottweilers, St. Bernards and Staffordshire Terriers are considered to have barrel-shaped chests.

Bird dogs refer to any dog used by man for hunting.

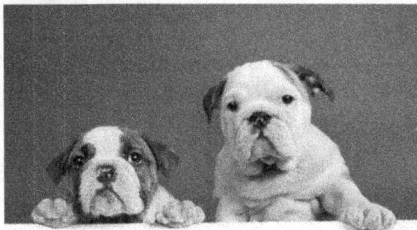

Brachycephalic or flat-faced dogs have a broad, short head with a pushed-in face. Special care should be taken as these dogs often suffer breathing difficulties due to their shortened nasal passages. Do not let them get overweight or overheated as distress can occur quickly. The Boston Terrier, Boxer, English and French

Bulldogs belong to this group while the Brussels Griffon, Cavalier King Charles, Pekingese, Pug, Shih Tzu and Yorkshire Terrier are often referred to as Extreme Brachycephalic meaning their muzzle practically disappears into the face.

Detection dogs are trained to detect explosives, drugs, food items, dead bodies and even human illness, while Guide Dogs assist blind, deaf and immobile humans by serving as their non-functioning eyes, ears and limbs.

Dogs with an elliptical shaped chest (such as the Jack or Parsons Russell) have a longer more flattened rib cage which can compress slightly allowing them to go underground or in tighter quarters while maintaining sufficient lung capacity.

Lap dogs fit into your lap for cuddling; however, a 75 pound dog can become a lap dog at the sound of a loud noise so don't rule any canine out of this category.

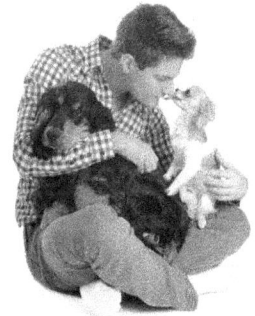

Molossoid dogs have deep wide chests and blunt muzzles such as the Mastiff, Bulldog, Cane Corso, Dogue de Bordeaux, Presa Canario, Rottweiler and Sharpei.

Non-Shedding is a deceiving term as every dog sheds some hair and dander, but some shed way more than others. Breeds that shed minimally include the Affenpinscher, Airedale, American Hairless Terrier, Basenji, Bichon, Cairn Terrier, Chinese Crested, Doberman Pinscher, Havanese, Italian Greyhound, Maltese, Portuguese Water Dog, Puli, Shih Tzu, Soft-Coated Wheaton Terrier, Poodle and the Yorkie.

Scent hounds specialize in following a smell or scent. Their long drooping ears help them collect scent from the air and keep it near their face and nose. A few scent hounds include the Basset Hound, Beagle, Bloodhound, Dachshund, Foxhound, Norwegian Elkhound and Rhodesian Ridgeback.

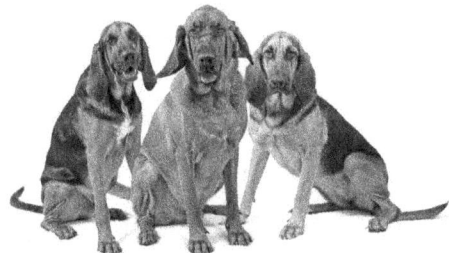

Sight or gazehounds have keen vision and great agility that helps them pursue prey by keeping it in sight and then overcoming it with tremendous speed. The Greyhound and Whippet may first come to mind, but the Afghan, Borzoi, Irish Wolfhound, Saluki and Scottish Deerhound are also this type.

Slab-sided or flat-ribbed dogs have a chest that is deeper at the midpoint making it the most flexible and compressible. Sighthounds are usually slab-sided which explains their ability to run long distances due to the flattened rib cage allowing the maximum intake of oxygen.

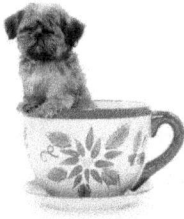

Teacup is a marketing term for Toy dogs. These dogs are mostly a result of selective breeding and include the Affenpinscher, Bichon Frise, Cairn Terrier, Chihuahua, American Hairless Terrier (but also comes in a larger size), Havanese, Maltese and Yorkshire Terriers.

Truffle Hounds are dogs that have been trained to find -- but not eat -- the high-priced truffles that grow underground.

In summary, there are a lot of types to choose from. Be sure to choose the pet that is best for you and your lifestyle.

Ask yourself:
- How much time can you spend with your dog each day?
- Where will your dog be while you are at work, school or running errands? In a crate, one room or have free roam of the house?
- Do you have a securely fenced yard for dogs that can jump over or dig under? Some canines are Houdinis and can escape just when you think you've covered all of your bases.
- Where will you place the dog's bed, bowls and toys so that they are not in the way but safely positioned?
- Can your budget accommodate an animal's basic needs? Food, bed, collar & leash, toys, micro-chipping, spay/neuter, veterinary exams, flea/tick prevention, training and the unexpected.
- How much time can you spend grooming? Even with a groomer, you need to do daily maintenance and a good head-to-tail check-up weekly (see page 42)!
- Will you be able to take care of your new best friend no matter what? If you move, add another family member (young or old), get a new job, go off to college, have a change in health or income, what will happen to your four legged family member?

Other Considerations:

Apartment Dweller?

Small dogs work well in small spaces, but retired Greyhounds can be couch potatoes and may be just as good of a choice as Pomeranians, Shih Tzus, Pugs, Bichon Frises and Terriers. Remember again, if your dog is going to be left alone, he may call out for you during the day, so a howler, barker or yapper may not be the best choice if you share walls with a neighbor.

Landlord Restrictions?

It doesn't have to be just an apartment...find out if your landlord allows pets and if there are specific restrictions (certain breeds, dogs under 30 lbs., etc.). You may be charged an additional fee but having a dog makes it all worthwhile. You must find out the details in advance, however, because if you bring home a 10 pound puppy that will be 80 pounds when full grown, or a breed not specifically agreed upon, you may end up having to move ('cause you certainly wouldn't give up that dog once you offered it a forever home now, would you?).

Local Laws?

Some jurisdictions only allow a certain number of pets per household (a combination of three dogs and/or cats for instance), so check with your local animal control before you adopt. Unfortunately, some cities ban specific breeds. Others may place restrictions on them (such as they must be spayed/neutered, wear a muzzle when in public or cannot roam certain areas). You are not only your dog's advocate, but you are also his protector and must know how to keep him safe as well as law-abiding.

Yard/Fencing?

The number of pets hit by cars every year is staggering. There are no guarantees, but teaching your dog to walk by your side on a leash with a properly fitting collar is about as close as you can come. Basic obedience training is a must, and combined with a well-secured fenced yard, it can literally save your dog's life.

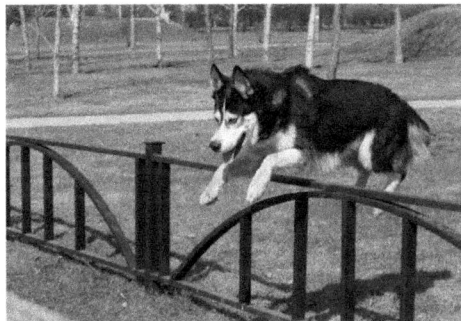

Dogs that don't roam the neighborhood also avoid:
- Pesticides on your neighbor's lawn
- Poisons in garbage cans
- Fights with other animals

When in that fenced yard, it is your responsibility to make sure your dog has access to shade, fresh water and time spent with you as well as an all-around safe environment to sniff the air or chase a squirrel. Take note at different times of the day and different seasons of the year to make sure the water bowl isn't in the scorching sun when your dog needs it most or that the shade cast by your tree isn't on the other side of the fence in the neighbor's yard late afternoon.

Some dogs can easily scale a six-foot wall or fence, so know your breed and your particular dog's athletic abilities to keep him safely contained in your yard. Big or small, dogs can dig and get themselves under and out of fencing, so you may need to pour a cement barrier under the fence line or line it with railroad ties or other materials to prevent an escape! Fence topping known as "coyote rollers" which keeps wildlife from hopping your fence may also prevent Fido from leaving.

Children?

Labrador Retrievers, Golden Retrievers, Shepherds and Schnauzers are only a few breeds that make wonderful family dogs while small dogs can sometimes become overwhelmed by the smallest humans and act snippy. Supervise ALL animals around children, and teach children not to disturb a dog while it is sleeping, eating or playing with its toys.

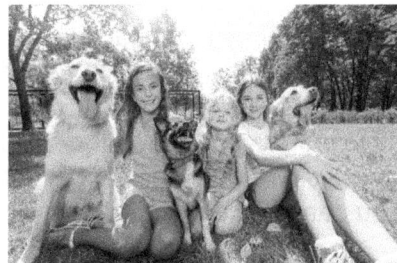

Both children and pets can be unpredictable and leaving them alone together without adult supervision could be a recipe for disaster. You must take charge and be there to intercede rather than trusting an animal or child to always do the right thing.

Allergies to Pets?

Don't rule out adding a dog to the family. Being around pets can strengthen the immune system (See "Zooeyia" later on this page), but check with your physician to see if there are medications to keep you comfortable should you get watery eyes, a runny nose or a case of the sneezes. Give it time, but vacuum the house regularly and bathe the dog weekly. All dogs shed but some that do so minimally include the Airdale, Bichon, Cairn Terrier, Maltese, Portuguese Water Dog, Puli, Shi Tzu, Poodle and Yorkie.

Other Pets?

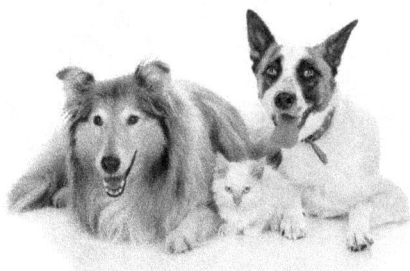

Introduce your dog slowly and carefully to other animals in the household. Just because you want one big happy family doesn't mean all animals will immediately (or ever) get along. Provide an out-of-claws-reach location for pocket pets, fish and birds which look like prey animals to many canines.

If you're considering adding a dog to your CANINE PACK... there just are no hard and fast rules. However, some breeds prefer not to share their lives with dogs of the same gender, so male-female combos often work best, but spay your female and neuter your male! The next best choice may be a male-male combo as female-female pairings can work but are the most likely to result in conflict.

Again, pay attention to individual personalities and activity levels -- an old tired dog may not enjoy a rambunctious young whipper-snapper, and then again...that puppy might be a breath of fresh air to the senior, egging him along to enjoy his second puppyhood. Know your dog. Observe your dog and let him meet the new comer on neutral turf before you make a commitment to make an addition to the family. See page 36 for tips on safely adding a new member to your pack.

Zooeyia?

Are you tilting your head like a confused canine about now? Zooeyia (ZOO-ey-ah) is a relatively new word which describes the health benefits pets provide us humans! It comes from the Greek roots "zoion" for animal and "Hygeia" for the Greek goddess of health, and its inventors consider it the opposite of Zoonosis which you'll read about on page 55. Zoonosis refers to diseases that can be transferred between species, meaning ones you can get from your pets.

Science is proving that making a pet part of your family can decrease the risk of developing colds and asthma by developing stronger immune systems. Pets lower our stress and also our blood pressure, but there are other health issues recently identified by the Institute of Medicine of the National Academies:

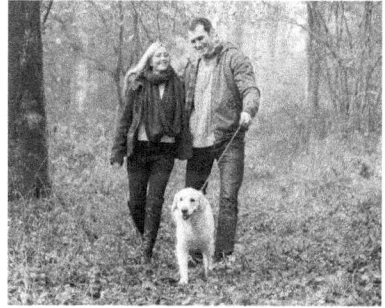

- Canine best friends get us moving. Humans of all ages with dogs in the family exercise more than those who do not share their lives with a dog as the dog's need for walks gets us up and going too.
- Pets lower the impact of chronic disease. Studies have shown pets decrease the risk of cardiovascular disease in their owners. Having a pet in the life of a cancer patient has been shown to provide comfort and support during treatment, which can decrease stress and releases endorphins.
- Pets help us kick the habit. Research has shown that knowing secondhand smoke can harm our pets has motivated some smokers to quit!
- Dogs make us more social. Loneliness and isolation can occur in our increasingly urbanized lifestyles, especially among the elderly. Having a pet gets us out meeting people, taking part in activities with other pet parents, going to parks, hiking and just staying in touch with the world.

Do your research, and make a well thought out decision before you adopt, and then embrace the joys of having a pet as part of the family! Not only will you have a furry friend who loves you unconditionally, but also look at all the other ways he may benefit your health as well.

WHERE TO MEET YOUR NEW DOG?

Local Animal Shelters take in 3 - 4 million dogs and cats each year. A common myth is that shelters only have mixed breeds, but it is simply not true! In most cases, 25% are purebreds, and the rest are amazing animals too. Visit several times and spend time interacting with the dog before deciding. Do not choose through a window or kennel door alone. Many humans feel that rescue pets are particularly grateful for being saved, but if you are looking for a specific breed that you can't find at your local shelter, breed-specific rescue organizations can be found on-line.

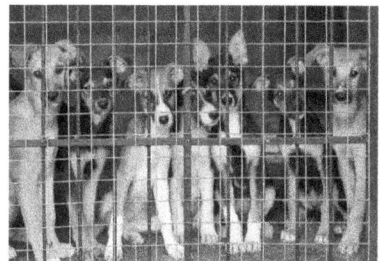

Responsible breeders take their jobs of raising dogs seriously. You'll know they are responsible not only by the care given and the depth of their knowledge, but they also will agree to take back the animal at any time during his life if you are unable to care for him. To locate a responsible breeder, contact the American Kennel Club (AKC), or other reputable organization.

At all costs, avoid stores that sell puppy mill pets. Puppy mills are factory farms where breeding moms suffer horrific atrocities. Many have never felt grass under their paws or have left their wire cages. When buying from a pet store, if you do your research, you might find that the mom of the adorable pup you're considering is spending her life in misery cranking out litter after litter until she can't anymore. More and more pet stores across the country are jumping on the bandwagon inviting rescue groups to adopt at their stores rather than selling puppy mill pets.

SATISFYING YOUR DOG'S BASIC NEEDS

Get off on the right paw with your new best friend by fulfilling his basic needs for a longer, happier lifetime together:

1) Quality Time Spent with You
2) Supplies
3) Health & Safety Team
4) Identification
5) Nutrition
6) Exercise & Stretching, Socialization & Basic Manners
7) Educate yourself for your pet's sake

1) Quality Time Spent with YOU

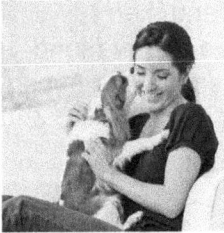

The true meaning of life for your dog is quality time spent with their favorite person -- YOU! Canine lives are much shorter than ours, so make every minute count and live in the moment with your precious pet. Take time out to do special activities together, such as throwing a ball, grooming, belly rubs & ear scratches, hiking or getting involved in agility (cats too are now taking up this sport), nose-work, or chasing a feather -- whatever makes you smile and your dog wag!

2) Supplies
- Bed
- Bowls
- Brush, Comb, Flea Comb
- Carrier/Crate
- Collar, Leash & Car Restraints
- Dog License
- Flea & Tick Prevention
- Food
- Pet Toothbrush & Pet Specific Toothpaste
- ID Tag that is clearly legible & Microchip properly registered & maintained
- Necessary medication/supplements
- Pet First-Aid Kit
- Pet Sitter when you can't be there
- Plan for their care if you are injured
- Toys
- Training
- Veterinary Care/Insurance

3) Your Dog's Health & Safety Team (aka their body guards, entourage, people)

Through research and conversation with other pet parents and professionals, you must assemble a team to care for your pet. The primary caregivers, also known as your pet's 'second best friends' (well you are #1 after all), should include your Veterinarian, Emergency Center Personnel, Obedience Trainer for dogs, Groomer and Pet Sitter. You could need to add to the team depending on your lifestyle or pet's needs, so those humans may include: Boarding or Daycare Staff, Dog Walker, Animal Behaviorist, Animal Communicator, Holistic Veterinarian, Massage Therapist, Acupuncturist and/or Nutritionist along with various medical specialists. Additionally, you should designate at least 2-3 people who could care for your dog in the event you are unable to and have paper work in order to make sure your wishes are honored. (See form on page 237).

Veterinarian

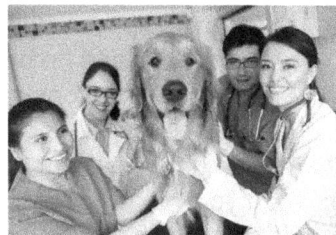

Consider your Veterinarian's qualifications, but also:
- Location, office hours, payment options, range of services
- Can you get an appointment quickly?
- Is your Veterinarian's philosophy and openness to alternative treatments in line with your own beliefs?
- Does the Veterinarian have a good bedside manner and answer questions to your satisfaction? Knowledge and expertise is a wonderful thing, but since you speak or your dog who cannot, you must put together a team of humans that YOU and your pet can relate to and build a good rapport with.

Ask friends if they like their Veterinarian and notice:
- If the office is clean
- If the waiting room accommodates multiple pets
- If the front office staff is helpful and tends to stay
- If they are a member of the American Animal Hospital Association (AAHA) which means they have met certain standards.
- If they are Fear Free® Certified; meaning they will do their best for your pet's stress as well as his health.
- The office environment and the interactions of staff, noting if people and pets are treated in a manner you are comfortable with, if there are safe waiting areas and if the general care and vibe fits your needs.

Bring your pet to the Veterinarian for
- Annual check-ups
- Vaccinations
- Spay/Neuter - Unaltered pets roam in search of a mate and 80% of animals killed on highways are non-neutered males. Animals that aren't "fixed" often display a higher level of aggression and are at greater risk for pyometra, mammary and prostate cancers. With 3 - 4 million homeless animals being euthanized each year, become part of the solution, not part of the problem.
- Senior exams including blood panel and urinalysis
- Anytime your dog is not quite right.

Animal Emergency Center

Some are open 24/7 while others keep the hours your Veterinarian is closed…6pm – 8am the next morning. Find the one nearest your home, your favorite park or hiking location and wherever your dog goes and DRIVE THERE! Writing down the address and phone number is not enough. When an emergency happens you must be on auto-pilot and know where you are headed for your pet's sake.

Must Know:
- Where the office is located
- Where to park
- What entrance you will bring your dog in (If you have a 100 lbs. dog that can't walk, this can be of major importance)
- What services can be provided – Is the facility equipped for x-rays, MRIs, transfusions, surgeries? Do they carry antivenin for snake bites? Do your research and be prepared before you need to help your pet.
- Payment options

Whether an emergency or routine care, veterinary insurance could help you help your pet when your bank account cannot. Check into the various options and restrictions, researching which plan is best for you and the current dog in your life. Deductibles and procedures covered vary from policy to policy. Should you opt not to purchase insurance, you may be preventing your pet from getting much-needed care, so have a Plan B! At the very least, have an emergency credit card or a separate bank account that you contribute to monthly in the event your furry loved one needs medical care.

Dog Obedience Trainer

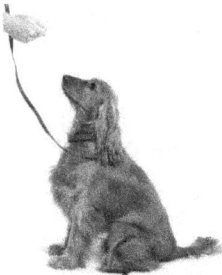

Every dog needs manners and someone to teach them to him! If hiring a professional dog obedience trainer isn't in your budget, you must then take the time to learn to speak dog by educating yourself and then paying attention to your pooch. There are many ways to train but you need to make an intelligent or educated decision about which method is best for your individual dog. In the long run, spending money on a professional trainer often outweighs money spent repairing items a destructive pet may have destroyed or the hospital bills incurred when your dog hasn't learned to not run into traffic or has consumed something hazardous. All dogs do not need to run circles between your feet, balance a cookie on his snout or sneeze on command, but ALL dogs need to learn basic obedience to become welcomed members of the family! "Come" can help your dog stay out of harm's way. "Sit" means "please" in doggie terms while "Leave it" could prevent him from ingesting poison! Humans have boundaries and do best when courteous so our four-legged companions must be taught to do the same for a happy and safe lifetime together.

Ask your friends, Veterinarian, groomer, local pet store and surf the internet. Finding the right Obedience Trainer may require you to observe several classes as each uses different techniques and methods.

You then must work consistently with your dog EVERY DAY, several times in short 5 - 10 minute sessions. Repetition is key. Don't expect to take your dog to a six-week class / one-hour per week and have him trained. Learning takes place on a daily basis at home with you and continues throughout his lifetime. You CAN teach an old dog (or a puppy) new tricks and especially manners and should continue to do so to keep his mind sharp and you engaged in his life.

Groomer

Most people think of this team member as the beautician, but there is much more to a groomer than the fur on your cat or dog! The groomer, even more than your Veterinarian, gets down to your pet's skin and can notice eruptions, cuts, scrapes, allergies and rashes. Your groomer may find a bump while bathing your cat or notice your dog's ears are infected. Choose your groomer well, and he or she may be your pet's first line of defense in finding a problem before it becomes a nightmare.

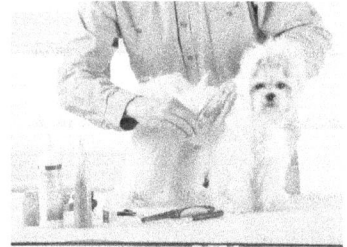

Pet Sitter

Although the enthusiastic neighboorhood teen who loves your dog or cat may be a good choice to watch him or her when you're away, please hire a professional pet sitter for your fur kid. The person caring for your best friend must take the responsibility to heart and seriously prepare to handle whatever life throws their way when caring for a precious life. Your pet's sitter should be licensed, bonded and able to anticipate a situation BEFORE it arises with the confidence to handle it. Yes, you want a true blue animal person who will greet your pet, maybe even before he or she greets you, but also one who can read animal body language and observe mood changes. You also need someone who can carefully place kitty in and out of her carrier, administer medications or divert an incident with other dogs when out walking yours. Someone who will follow your directions to a tee and check twice that your dog's harness is securely fastened. Knowledge, experience and dependability are key traits to seek out in your pet's caregiver.

Just as you are learning from this book, a professional pet sitter keeps on learning better ways to relate to and care for animals, can safely administer Pet First-Aid & CPCR and must know what to do if the power goes out or a pipe breaks when you are away -- For your pet's sake. A professional pet sitter prides him or herself on staying current on all things pet -- the latest in nutrition, exercise, safety and care, so they are an excellent resource for you as well. Seeking a recommendation from other conscientious pet parents or your Veterinarian (many Vet techs pet sit on the side) is a GRRReat choice, but professional organizations, such as Pet Sitters International™, can provide you with a list of certified professional pet sitters in your area. PSI and NAPPS (National Association of Professional Pet Sitters) provide on-line and in-person trainings to their members, provide excellent guidelines to keep them organized with their sits and motivate them to be the best pet caregiver they can be.

Once you have chosen a reliable pet sitter, make sure you put into place any authorizations needed on your pet's behalf, so that the pet sitter may obtain necessary care for your dog or cat in your absence. Put everything in writing that your pet's caregiver should know including medical history, food, places pet sleeps and hide. Fill in your Pet's Health Record on page 247, and you'll be set. Talk with your Veterinarian's office to determine if a letter is required (and possibly your credit card) to be kept on file to allow your pet sitter to make medical decisions for your pet if you are not reachable. Discuss this also with your pet sitter, so that he or she knows to what extent you want medical care for your pets and who you want providing treatment for them.

You – The Pet Guardian

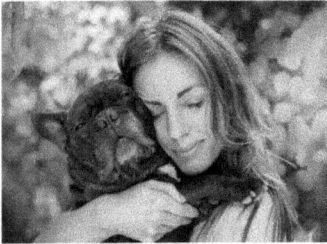

Tune in to your pet every day to notice subtle changes and stay in-the-know to get the latest information on how you can help your pet live a longer, happier healthier life! Don't be on the cell phone when walking Fido or watching TV while playing with Fluffy - give them your undivided attention for at least 20 minutes each day and even more time just spent near or with you.

Be proactive and don't wait for tragedy to strike. Keep a simple Identification Card (like you'll find on page 257) in your wallet to let first responders know you have pets at home that need caring for if something happens to you. Can you imagine your poor dogs trying to "hold it" for days or wondering when you'll be home to feed them if you haven't made this plan? Besides filling out the paperwork, you MUST be sure that caregivers you designate are totally on board and know how you'd like your pet cared for. Include funds for them to do so. Hopefully this care will just be short term, but it is wise to meet with an attorney and put everything in writing. Publish this document, making sure others know it exists and that these are your wishes. This should NOT be part of your Will as it could need to be enacted while you are still alive, such as if you are in a coma or suffer some other disability that will not permit you to care for your best friends. Don't let your fur kids be relinquished or sent off to a Shelter because you didn't take the time to plan for them. You can't assume family members will make them their own. Get everything legally prepared and confirm with all parties involved. Also designate at least three caregivers as circumstances in their own lives may have changed when they are needed most.

4) <u>Identification Should Include</u>
   - Dog's name
   - Your name, address, telephone numbers
   - Medical problem(s) requiring medication
   - Veterinarian's name & number
   - Current rabies vaccination information
   - Reward offer which increases chances your dog will be returned to you

Microchips are important as tags can fall off. A microchip is a tiny electronic chip enclosed in a glass cylinder (about the size of a grain of rice) that is injected just under your pet's skin – between his shoulder blades – with a hypodermic needle. The microchip does not have a battery but is activated when a scanner is passed over your pet. It transmits an ID number to the scanner along with the name of the microchip's manufacturer. If you have done your homework and sent the registering agency your contact information, your pet's microchip will identify them as belonging to you.

Microchips are a safe and effective way to reunite pets with their humans – they are also used on cats, birds, horses, rabbits, and just about any pet.

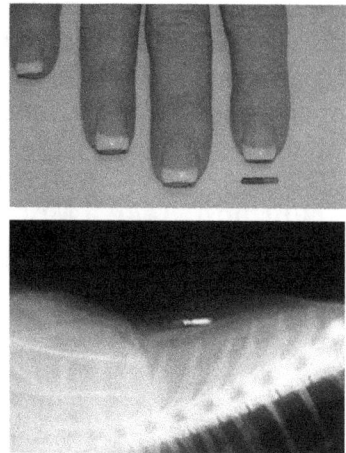

Photos by Sunny-dog Ink

Check tags regularly to insure information is legible and accurate.

The friction resulting from your pet's tags clanging together during the normal course of each day causes the engraving to rub off or become difficult to read. Check your pet's tags regularly to determine if they can be easily read. Also have your dog scanned during his annual veterinary visit to make sure the microchip is still in place (they can migrate in your pet's body) and working as it should. Update contact information with your microchip company when you move or change a phone number, and check with your local animal shelter to make sure they use a universal scanner that reads your microchip. If not, encourage them to get one that does or make sure your pets have microchips that can be read by your local facility.

Good to Know:

The International Standards Organization (ISO) has approved a global standard for microchips which is intended to create a consistent ID system worldwide. For example, if your dog or cat is implanted with an ISO standard microchip in the U.S. travels to Europe with you and becomes lost, the ISO standard scanners in Europe would be able to read the microchip. If your dog however was implanted with a non-ISO microchip, it might not be detected or be read by the scanner.
Should your pet ever go missing:

Contact your microchip company, Veterinarian and local shelter at once, and quickly go to places that are familiar to your pet – dog parks, neighbors' homes your pet visits, favorite water hole or where he sits while you sip your morning coffee.

Make flyers using a current photo and stating a reward (it definitely increases the chances of re-uniting you with your best friend) and circulate them all over the neighborhood taking care to abide by city rules as to where and how you may post. Walk the neighborhood asking if anyone has seen your dog and visit local shelters as well as various websites with data bases that list found pets.

Hire one of the many services out there that will make robo-calls to your entire neighborhood and get your pet's photo on numerous websites and social media to increase the possibility of a safe return. There are trained Pet Detectives, some even use dogs to find your pet, so get acquainted with the various help available to help your pet find his way home. ("Missing Pet" flyer template on page 236)

5) <u>Nutrition: Take a More Active Role in Your Dog's Diet and Health by Choosing the Best Food for Your Dog</u>

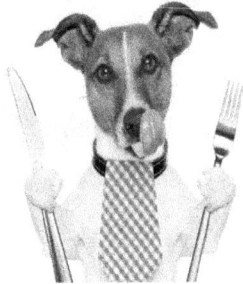

"You are what you eat." Although this phrase has a contrived history dating back centuries, it didn't emerge in English until 1940 when nutritionist Victor Lindlahr wrote the book so entitled expressing his strong belief that food controls health. It holds true for our canine friends too.

Most consumers are unaware that the pet food industry got its early start as an opportunity to sell off waste from the human food industry. Shocking but true, contaminated and low quality sources of meat (animal by-products) that are rejected by the USDA (United States Department of Agriculture) can be sold to pet food companies at bargain prices. These discarded ingredients may include intestines, udders, heads, hooves and even diseased and cancerous animal parts. But there is good news! "Fortunately, more progressive pet food companies are rejecting the use of inferior meat and grain by-products, are accepting only USDA-inspected meats, and are not adding artificial flavorings and unnatural preservatives to their new diets," says Paula Terifaj, DVM in Brea, California. Therefore, one of the best things you can do for your dog is to know what you are feeding him. To do so you must read and understand pet food labels and research the brand you buy.

BCDF (Before Commercial Dog Food)

Less than a hundred years ago, the family pet ate leftovers and table scraps in addition to scavenging and hunting. Whether dogs truly thrived on this diet is hard to say according to Deb Eldredge, DVM in Vernon, New York. "We keep better records now and have better diagnostics."

INCREASED AWARENESS

The move towards healthier eating by people shows in the concern over our dog's diet as well. Susan Blake Davis, a Certified Clinical Nutritionist who provides holistic pet health consultations nationwide claims, "Many health-minded pet owners want the same high quality food for their pets that they eat themselves. While many are preparing homemade foods, others are demanding that the same quality be found in commercially prepared foods that are convenient and easy to use. As a result, there are lots of wonderful brands on the market." However, Dr. Terifaj cautions not to be fooled by claims that pet foods labeled 'balanced and nutritionally complete' really are. "You are in a dangerous comfort zone if you believe that any one diet can be formulated [to be complete for every pet.]"

Each dog, like every individual human, is different with varying genetics, environments, sensitivities and needs. No one diet is perfect for all. Dogs out of the same litter may not thrive on the same diet.

Additionally, the Menu Foods Recall of 2007 brought to light the fact that store bought pet food isn't always safe and can be life-threatening. "With commercially prepared food," explains Dr. Eldredge, "dogs are now getting a more balanced diet. In the past Veterinarians saw more cases of vitamin deficiencies or excesses, yet on the other hand, with the mass production of food, if a contaminated ingredient gets into the diet, we have large numbers of dogs throughout a wide area being affected."

The 2007 Recall wasn't the first but it was the largest. In 1998 fifty-three brands of pet food were found to be contaminated with aflatoxin (a toxin produced by mold that can damage the liver) and ten more brands in 2005. There were other recalls prior and more have and will follow, so pet parents need to take a more active role in the health of their pets.

Ignore packaging and clever names. Look at the actual ingredients. Much of the commercial food available today is made for the benefit of the consumer. It is made to be convenient, colorful and attractive. Orange carrot-shaped treats give consumers the false sense that they are giving their pet a real carrot. Remember that Mother Nature gives us our most basic rules: *Eat fresh, choose variety and buy wholesome.*

Must-know Vocabulary as determined by the AAFCO (Association of American Food Control Officials)…

Meat is "the clean flesh derived from slaughtered mammals and is limited to that part of the striate muscle which is skeletal or that which is found in the tongue, diaphragm, heart or esophagus."

Poultry is "the clean combination of flesh and skin with or without accompanying bone, derived from the parts or whole carcasses of poultry or a combination thereof, exclusive of feathers, heads, feet and entrails."

Meal is the rendered product from mammal tissues, exclusive of any added blood, hair, feathers, hooves, horn, hide, trimmings, manure, stomach and rumen contents except in such amounts as may occur unavoidably."

By Product consists of "non-rendered clean parts of carcasses free from fecal content and foreign matter."

MBM aka Meat and Bone Meal is a catch-all term where the worst stories come from about pet food. Some renderers accept road kill, euthanized pets, animals who died on farms, during transport, fetuses and out-of-date supermarket meat so MBM is a signal that the food is of inferior quality for your best friend.

Basic Guidelines:

- The first two ingredients should be whole sources of specific animal protein: beef, chicken, lamb, salmon, venison, turkey or other animal protein...The name of the animal in the bag or can. Stay away from the terms "meat," "poultry" and "fish" which are too vague.
- Whenever possible limit or avoid meat & filler by-products as well as fillers (wheat, corn and soy for instance which can cause allergies or are hard for pets to process).
- Stay away from food dyes, sweeteners such as propylene glycol and sorbitol, additives like smoke or beef flavor and sodium nitrite which all carry health risks.
- As a rule, canned food is preferable to dry for cats as they suffer less urinary tract and kidney problems when consuming food that has water in it.
- Avoid artificial preservatives (BHA, BHT and ethoxyquin), and seek out foods using natural antioxidants like vitamins C, E and mixed tocopherols. Frozen foods avoid the use of unnatural preservatives altogether since freezing naturally preserves food.
- Educate yourself as to which human foods are unsafe for your pet. Two good sources are www.aspca.org and www.hsus.org.

The best diet for any pet is the diet that pet does best on. This will vary even within a breed as well as by age, gender and activity level. An adult dog for instance does not need as much calcium as a puppy or lactating female. Since dogs have been bred for different purposes throughout different parts of the world, various breeds have dietary needs and require staple ingredients that can be traced back to their beginnings. German Shepherds have small colons and often do better on a diet high in fiber to slow the movement of food, giving the body more time to absorb the nutrients it needs while Labrador Retrievers generally do not digest beef, corn or soy properly. Golden Retrievers have a hard time digesting ocean fish, soy and white rice. Knowing genetic problems that are common in certain breeds can help determine proper nutrition and help prevent health issues from arising.

Pay attention to the sparkle in your pet's eyes, his energy level, coat condition and passion for life. Have him tested for any deficiencies or diseases that could be improved by a proper diet. A few more dollars spent on more nutritious food can reduce veterinary visits and improve the health of your four-legged best friend. That is truly priceless!

Label Reading 101

There's no way around it. To be a responsible pet parent, you must learn to read pet food labels to avoid buying an inferior product for your canine best friend. Some higher priced foods also contain undesirable ingredients, so don't be fooled by the price tag or marketing campaign. Clever advertising gurus try to seduce you with photos of succulent meats and vegetables and happy animal faces. Don't judge any pet food by its wrapper!

Ingredients are listed in descending order of weight, and animal protein is the single most important ingredient in pet food, so look at the first few ingredients listed to determine the main sources of protein being used. Pay attention if other items are broken into components -- if chicken is listed first, but then comes corn gluten, corn meal and ground corn, those three corn components may add up to a higher concentration than the chicken.

Equally important as what you want to see on the label, are those items you do not want to see – chemical additives and preservatives. Below is a brief glossary of labeling "buzz" words to familiarize yourself with:

All or 100% cannot be used (according to AAFCO guidelines) "if the product contains more than one ingredient, not including water sufficient for processing, [includes anything that colors substandard meats to look more natural], or trace amounts of preservatives and condiments]."

95% Rule applies when the ingredients derived from animals, poultry or fish make up 95% or more of the total weight of the product (or 70% excluding water for processing).

Flavor means the ingredients impart a distinctive characteristic to the food. Therefore, a "beef flavor" food may contain a small quantity of digest (material which results from a chemical or enzymatic process) or other extract of tissues or artificial flavor, without containing any actual beef meat at all.

Guaranteed analysis provides a very general guide to the composition of the food. Crude protein, fat, fiber and total moisture are required to be listed. Beware that the term crude protein allows pet food manufacturers to include items such as feathers, hair, hooves, tendons, and ligaments in their diets. While these animal by-products certainly contain protein, they are essentially indigestible and provide no nutritional value to your dog.

Holistic has yet to be embraced by regulations and standards with regards to pet food, so any manufacturer can claim the phrase on their packaging.

Human grade can be misleading unless the entire product is edible by humans, in accordance to USDA and FDA standards.

Organic means USDA rules and regulations must be followed and the product will have the USDA organic seal on the packaging.

Natural does not have an official definition but is construed to mean the product does not contain artificial flavors, artificial colors or artificial preservatives.

Premium, Super Premium, Ultra Premium and Gourmet labeled foods are not required to contain higher quality ingredients, nor are they held to higher nutritional standards than are any other product.

With, such as "with real chicken," means that ingredient accounts for at least 3% of the food by weight, excluding water for processing.

Pet health experts see a definite trend towards home pet food preparation – whether completely from scratch or by adding to a base commercial diet. There are some basic diets now sold with the intention of having meat or eggs added to balance them. Many dogs enjoy a bit of yogurt (if they aren't lactose-intolerant) or ground turkey added to their kibble.

When adding raw vegetables to a meal, throwing the greens into a food processor to break down the cellulose (the cell wall of green plants) can help your pet absorb the nutrients, but "wash them first!" And avoid onions, raisins, grapes, avocado and macadamia nuts, all of which can be toxic to your pets (see common poisons page 235).

With the raw food market continuing to expand as well as the arrival of packaged fresh frozen food (which does not require preservatives), it appears people are understanding the benefits and are getting back to basics for the health of their dogs.

Regardless of your choice, educate yourself on canine nutrition, practice proper hygiene and pay attention to how your pet responds to his food. Allergic reactions can present themselves as upset stomachs (vomiting and/or diarrhea), gas or belching, itchy skin or odorous infections, bald patches, constant paw or tail chewing, low energy to lethargy, hyperactivity, pale gums, bright red gums, rapid heart rate or breathing as well as anything that is not right with your pet. Tune in to notice any changes in your furry kid, and then take action by discussing with your Veterinarian or pet nutritionist. Advancements continue and there are new tests on the market that are less invasive and don't require your pet to be injected with allergens. Some tests screen for an elevation in antibodies. This could alert your Veterinarian early – when your dog's body is just starting to react or become sensitive. A saliva analysis streamlines the necessity of doing lengthy food trials (where one ingredient at a time is eliminated from your pet's diet) and may help get your furry companion on the path to a diet better suited for him.

Supplements:

Puppies, dogs in the prime of their lives, and even our senior four-legged friends can benefit from supplements! Most pets just do not get proper vitamins, minerals and antioxidants in their diet, even when fed top-of-the-line food, so supplements can fill the gap. Commercial pet food sometimes contains by-products and useless fillers that can be toxic. Food with such ingredients can create unstable oxygen molecules - known as free radicals – which have been shown to cause a wide range of health problems including allergies, skin & coat problems, arthritis, tumors, cancer, cataracts, strokes and heart disease. Free radicals beat up the cells in our pet's bodies continuously throughout each day until they weaken the cells. Antioxidants are like super heroes dissolving these free radicals and protecting our pets. Another type of Supplement gaining popularity is Adaptogens. Adaptogens work with the body to read, repair and restore body system balance. Work with a pet herbal expert or holistic practitioner to choose the proper supplements for your pets and their particular needs.

Once on supplements, you may not notice any outward change if your pet appears healthy, but know that a quality supplement is working inside your dog's body helping to keep the cells strong and healthy.

Consult with a knowledgeable Veterinarian or pet nutritionist to determine your dog's individual dietary needs. Some may benefit from a multi, whereas others will need specific vitamins, minerals or herbal remedies (see page 127 on Homeopathy).

6) Exercise & Stretching, Socialization & Basic Manners

Exercise entertains your dog and keeps muscles toned, joints limber and weight under control. Some dogs may need to be tricked into exercising. Give your bundle of fur plenty of toys, interactive tools and play with them often. Make it fun!

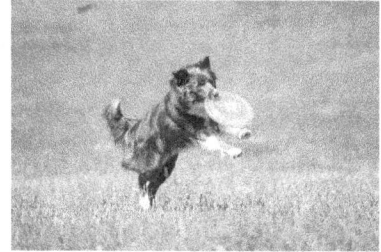

Physical activity and fresh air do a canine body good, and both are imperative for keeping your dog's body and mind sharp. Even as your dog gets older, continue to keep him moving at a pace determined by your Veterinarian as boredom is the playground for bad habits and destructive behaviors like digging which can lead to Houdini-like escapes. Don't use your fenced yard as a dog sitter. Dogs are task-oriented animals and need to keep busy. If you don't provide entertainment, they will find something to do!

Exercise ideas:

- Throw the ball/disc, brush your dog or teach him tricks.
- Take him for daily walks to provide a change of scenery to stimulate his brain as well as a cardio work-out.
- Enroll in group training classes, boot camp, agility/pulling/ herding/tracking classes depending on his breed and special abilities. There are even opportunities to dance with your dog.
- Teach your dog to swim with supervision.

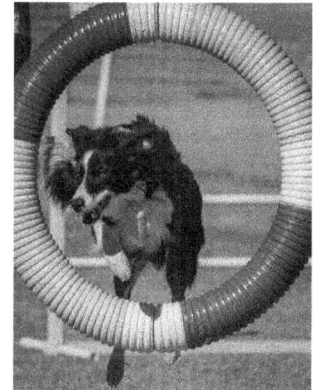

A tired dog is a good dog, and he'll reward you by settling down for a nap with a smile on his face.

Exercise may benefit your pet by:
- Lowering risks of arthritis, diabetes and other health related issues
- Keeping joints and ligaments limber and preventing muscle strains
- Delaying the loss of bone density
- Preventing muscles from atrophying
- Limiting weight gain
- Stimulating the brain

Stretching

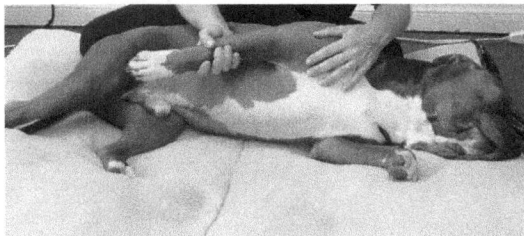

Photo Courtesy of Pam Holt.

Following exercise, stretch your pooch – slowly and gently to decrease pain, improve mobility and increase his range of motion preventing future injuries. Stretching can improve the longevity and wellness of any pet, not just the canine athlete.

This topic is a full volume on its own but areas to concentrate include the hips, shoulders and back. Done slowly and gently, most pets tolerate them well, however, if you feel uncertain, ask your Veterinarian, animal massage therapist or pet specific chiropractor to show you how.

Have your pet stand or lying on his side if he prefers, except for the chest, stretch when he's on his back, belly up! Some animals feel vulnerable in this position, so don't force him on his back if that is the case as you will negate the effects by creating stress. If your pet shows any sign of pain during stretching, stop what you are doing and make a veterinary appointment ASAP.

- Chest muscles endure a great deal of strain. To stretch this area your goal is to carefully and gently pull the muscles away from center. With your pet on his back (if he is agreeable to this), grasp both front legs near the wrists and gently open them out to the side. Hold for 5 seconds, release and repeat. Feel free to relax him further with circular massage strokes to his chest or belly while in this position.
- Shoulder flexors create smooth movement in your pet's front legs. It is best if your pet will stand. Hold his front leg above the elbow while placing your other hand underneath the elbow, stabilizing it. Gently stretch his leg forward as if doing a "high five." At the point of resistance, hold the position 15 - 30 seconds and repeat 2 - 3 times for each front leg.

Not only does this stretch improve the integrity of the shoulders, wrists and elbows, but it can also increase breathing capacity by loosening chest muscles allowing for lung expansion.

- Hip Flexors are the muscles that allow your cat or dog to move his legs and hips while walking or running. Best with your pet standing, hold his back leg above the knee, and gently stretch it straight back behind your pet's body. When you reach a point of resistance, where you'd actually be pulling the leg, stop and hold the position 15 - 30 seconds. Repeat 2 - 3 times with each back leg.

This stretch can increase flexibility in your pet's hips and spine while strengthening the lower back, hip and leg muscles. It may also lessen arthritis pain.

- Back stretching is a dog's favorite and it necessitates the use of treats! With your pet standing and you behind him or to one side, slowly move the treat from his nose towards his tail, encouraging your pet to follow with his eyes, only turning his head bending his body into a "C" shape. Make him hold the position for a count of 15 - 30 seconds, then repeat the exercise making the pet twist in the opposite direction. Do 2 - 3 stretches on each side. A good rub at the base of the tail, between the hip bones and up the spine feels especially good after this stretch. This helps increase the flow of spinal fluid and aids in the mobility of both your pet's hips and back.

Socializing:

Socializing goes hand-in-paw with obedience training. A well-socialized pet is friendly around other animals and people, is a welcome visitor to parks, pet-friendly locales and is an agreeable member of the family. He is less apt to get into a fight with other animals out of fear or bad manners.

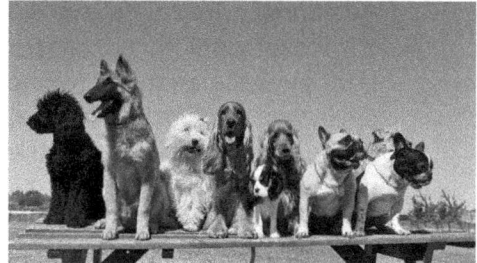

Start early and slowly:

- Introduce your dog to family members and friends. Have them make your dog sit and give him a treat.
- Desensitize your pets to sounds around the house…vacuum cleaner, stereo, clapping hands, the doorbell, and for cats…the neighboring dog's bark!
- Take your dog to a variety of places on-leash so he can see bicycles, skateboards, canes, wheel chairs and walkers and won't be startled by them.

Dog parks exist in many communities and can be an excellent way to improve your pooch's socialization skills. Dog park etiquette however, must be followed by both YOU and YOUR DOG in order to keep peace as well as humans and canines safe.

- Only bring dogs to a dog park that already have a history of getting along with other unfamiliar canines.
- Make sure your dog is spayed/neutered and current on all vaccinations as well as parasite preventives.
- Keep your dog on-leash until safely within the confines of the fencing.
- Abide by all rules which are often posted.
- If there are special areas for big dogs, small dogs, timid dogs, etc…only take your dog into the appropriate area.
- Bring your own water and bowl as community dog bowls can harbor germs.
- Pay attention to your dog at all times keeping him in sight and within grabbing distance. Too many humans use dog parks as human coffee klatch time and ignore the interaction taking place between the animals.
  - You cannot break up a fight or grab your dog if you have a hot cup of coffee in one hand.
  - If you're not paying attention to your dog and those near him, you won't be able to act quickly if needed.
- Keep a leash with you in the event you need to quickly lead your pet away or gain control of him.

- Know in advance where the nearest animal emergency center is in the event your dog sprains a leg, gets stung by a bee, bitten by a rattle snake or is on the receiving end of any injury.
- As the saying goes, leave every place cleaner than you found it. When at a dog park, make sure you take with you everything you brought or that you dog might leave behind. It is good etiquette. Doggie bags for waste clean-up are vital although many parks provide them or scoopers. Whatever the method – use it! Additionally, tennis balls or any toys you bring should go home with you. Not only will Rover want his possessions, but leaving them behind is a chance for disaster. If for instance a large dog finds the small ball or chew toy left behind by a Chihuahua or Cocker Spaniel. Too small for the larger mouth, the object could be found, swallowed and result in a choking incident possibly rendering the helpless pet unconscious. Don't be responsible for any animal being injured.

Basic Manners: Training

A well-behaved canine is less likely to escape into traffic or eat something he should not. An Obedience Trainer must be part of your dog's Health & Safety Team, but it is up to YOU to make sure that practice makes perfect. Money spent hiring a professional dog trainer will far outweigh damage resulting from a pet who has not learned his manners and who suffers injury from misbehaving.

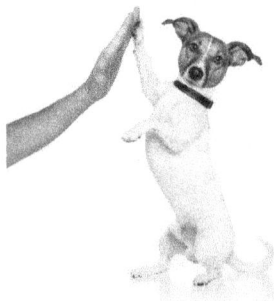

Have your dog achieve Canine Good Citizen® or similar status by passing a test administered through an instructor.

This will help you build a good foundation for having a well-mannered and well-qualified socialized dog. Skills your dog should excel at include:

- Accepting a friendly stranger
- Sitting politely for a petting
- Sitting nicely for grooming
- Walking on a loose lead
- Walking through a crowd politely and calmly
- Sit, down and stay in place
- Come when called
- Remaining calm in the presence of other dogs
- Remaining calm in the face of distractions (people, noises, wheelchairs, bicycles)
- Not becoming agitated or nervous when you are momentarily out-of-sight

Keep training sessions short (5-10 minutes at a time) and several times a day in the beginning until he has mastered each skill. Always use a happy voice and praise your dog ending each session on a good note – when your dog has accomplished something you can both be proud of. Release your dog from commands with 'Okay' or whatever word you choose and use consistently. However, choose a word you don't use often in conversation.

"HEEL" COMMAND
(aka Follow the Leader; the dog should be on your left and go where you go)

This is an excellent start to every training program in that it gets the dog moving and actually a bit tired physically and mentally as it requires him to think!

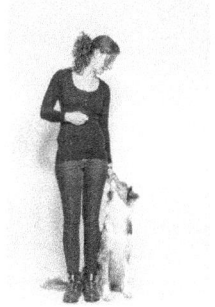

1) Start out with dog on your LEFT side, leash in your RIGHT hand and working
collar high up on the neck and under the dog's chin – just behind his ears. So as to move his head, not his esophagus or vocal chords.

2) Step off with your LEFT foot and walk with the dog by your left side.

3) If the dog tries to step in front of you, make a LEFT turn maneuvering him gently with your left knee to go in the direction YOU want. If he wanders ahead, give him a gentle tug on the leash (as if you're tapping someone on the shoulder and saying, "Hey buddy, where are you going?"), and reverse direction until the dog is back on your left following the leader.

4) PRAISE when he's doing well and keep moving until you feel you have the dog's attention.

*When training, YOU should be
THE most interesting thing to your dog.
His focus should be on YOU!*

"SIT" COMMAND (It's your pet's way of being polite and saying please)

"SIT" METHOD ONE
"Sit" means your dog is to sit on the spot.

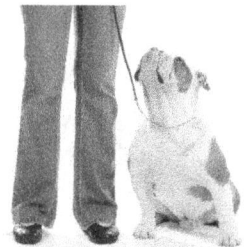

1) With the dog on your LEFT side, adjust working collar high up on the neck.

2) Hold leash in your RIGHT hand – don't give the dog too much slack which could allow him to move from your side.

3) As you give the command (elongate the "Siiiiiiiiit"), pull upward on the leash as you slide your left hand from the dog's neck to his rear encouraging him to move into the SIT position.

4) PRAISE with a happy voice!

"SIT" METHOD TWO

If a dog is shy or "rear" shy (meaning he doesn't like his back end touched), there is always another way.

1) Follow Steps 1 & 2 from previous.

2) Next, use a treat or toy to guide the dog to sit by slowly moving your hand with the item up over the dog's head. When his head raises, his rear end should lower.

3) PRAISE, praise, praise like there's no tomorrow, but just take care not to over-treat!

"STAY" COMMAND

"Stay" means your dog is not to move.

1) Once in the "Sit" position, use your flattened palm (like a "STOP" sign) in front of the dog's face.

2) If he moves, tell him "no," take him back to "Sit" and start over.

3) Once he stays, advance by trying to walk around him (keeping him on leash) and retaining the "Stay."

4) Don't forget PRAISE for a job well done!

NOTE: For all commands, keep collar high on neck for best control.

"COME" COMMAND

"Come" means to call the dog to you.

1) With dog on leash, change directions and call him to "come" to you, giving only a slight tug on the leash.

2) When he reaches you, praise.

"DOWN" COMMAND

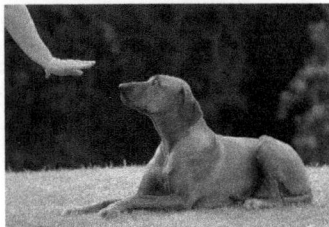

"Down" means you want the dog to lie down at your side. Do Not use this term, for instance, if you want your pet to "get down" from the couch or counter as will be confusing. Choose another word such as "Off" for that command.

1) As you slowly say "Down," place your LEFT hand on the leash near the collar and press in a downward motion until the dog is on all fours.

2) PRAISE for a job well done!

"LEAVE IT" COMMAND

'Leave It' means 'stop what you're doing' and can prevent your dog from consuming something he should not. It can also be used to teach your dog to ignore vehicles and moving objects. Use extra yummy treats to create more incentive.

1) Place an object (treat, toy, your slipper, etc.) in front of your dog while he is on-leash.

2) As he moves towards it, say "Leave it."

3) If he stops in his tracks, say "Good Dog," and treat him.

4) If not, pull back on his leash, make him sit and try again.

7) Educate Yourself and Don't Stop Learning for the Sake of Your Dog

There are so many opportunities these days to learn about animals - websites on every dog topic imaginable, webinars, YouTube videos, networks dedicated to animals, community college and classes at shelters, obedience training facilities and doggie day care centers. Libraries offer lectures and book readings as well as shelves full of books on the subject. Radio and video programming (Internet, satellite and old-fashioned radio waves) bring a plethora of dog experts into your car or living room. Tune in and turn on to the vast array of information available about dogs and cats. Just do something, and keep on doing it for the sake of your four-legged best friend.

MASSAGE & YOUR PET

Massage may be the oldest and simplest form of medical care, and it may also be one of the most effective.

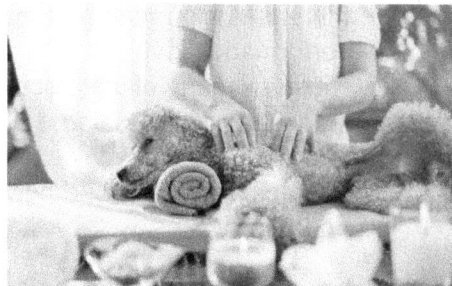

Egyptian tombs display drawings of humans being massaged while Chinese writings (circa 2,700 BC) recommend "breathing, massage of skin and... exercises of hands and feet" as the appropriate treatment for many ailments. Julius Caesar was said to have been given a daily massage to treat neuralgia. In the 5th Century BC, Hippocrates, the father of Western Medicine wrote, "The physician must be experienced in many things, but assuredly in rubbing...for rubbing can bind a joint that is too loose, and loosen a joint that is too rigid." So why not use massage to help our four-legged friends too?

Throughout history, massage has been used routinely on dogs and horses to aid and hasten recovery from injury, to provide relief from pain, and to calm and relax animals that live and work alongside humans. In the 21st Century, we are re-discovering the value of preventive care and recognizing the importance of viewing the body holistically. Our animal companions too are sharing the benefits as we implement natural and non-invasive modalities into their lives.

The power of massage comes from a focused touch. Basically, massage is touch with a purpose. According to Duke University Professor Dr. Saul Schanberg, "Touch is ten times stronger than verbal or emotional contact and is a key part to the survival of the animal species." In other words, touch is a biological need that affects almost every living creature!

Massage is the manipulation, methodical pressure, friction and kneading of the skin, muscle and soft tissues to achieve specific therapeutic results. Massage increases the flow of blood, nutrients and oxygen to all the tissues of the body which can accelerate the healing of an injury as well as the prevention of one by maintaining overall wellness. Injuries can be prevented by giving massage prior to heavy exercise and allowing your dog to warm-up and cool-down when participating in any type of sporting activity.

Massage for Injuries and Health

Massage therapy enhances every system of your dog's body – the immune, circulatory, endocrine, respiratory, nervous, digestive and lymphatic systems. Injury can be prevented if a pre-performance massage is given as muscles get warmed up with blood pumping through the tissues before activity begins.

Here are some additional benefits of massage:
- Stimulates the immune system which allows your dog to fight off infections.
- Increases the release of toxins from the body.
- Aids in the healing process.
- Lowers your dog's stress level and can have a calming effect on high-strung pets.
- Assists in training and competition as it creates focus.
- Increases the range and mobility of an animal's limbs thereby increasing their performance level.
- Relieves many of the discomforts of old age and degenerating conditions. Massage alleviates some of the pain and stiffness that comes with chronic arthritis and hip dysplasia.
- Creates a deeper bond between you and your pet while building confidence, trust and affection.

To **warm-up** your canine athlete, start with slow long continuous strokes (effleurage) from head to tail, down the outside and up the inside of limbs, gently increasing the pressure as you go. This will increase circulation, stretch the muscle fibers and warm the tissues.

Once you have warmed the muscles up, apply friction with your thumbs and fingers across the muscle fibers followed by the deeper petrissage. With your thumbs and fingers, gently knead and roll the skin improving oxygenation to the tissues. Begin lightly and increase pressure to release toxins and spasms from the muscles while bringing blood and nutrients to them. This is critical to their flexibility and movement for the competition ahead.

Conclude with more long strokes and gently stretch and flex your pooch by extending his limbs while always maintaining support of them. End the massage with more effleurage to clear the muscles of their metabolic waste.

To *cool-down* Fido after competition, use lots and lots of long strokes. Gently compress to drain the muscles of lactic acid that can be painful if allowed to build up. Since the muscles have been exerted during the course of exercise, use a lighter touch during your post-performance massage. Make slower and slower strokes as you attempt to cool the body down. Finish off with a cool refreshing bowl of water to aid in the elimination of toxins. Now pat your four-legged athlete on the back, give him a belly rub or ear scratch and enjoy the fond memories of competition and the thrill of having a healthy, happy dog!

In most instances, massage does not replace the need for surgery; however, for certain problems it can be quite beneficial. Massage and acupressure can help with muscle tension, spasms or knots commonly in the neck, back, shoulders and hind limbs that many canine athletes develop.

Massage and stretching can be very beneficial for dogs with hip dysplasia, cruciate or back surgery, but of course every animal is different. Massage and proper rehabilitation of a post-surgical anterior cruciate rupture may help prevent the need for surgery in the non-surgical leg. Most dogs, within a year's time, end up tearing the non-surgical ACL due to additional stress placed on it during recovery of the first leg.

Who Should Massage Your Pet?

Find someone who is certified in animal-specific massage therapy so that they're familiar with the anatomy and physiology of your pet. Like with your Veterinarian, groomer or anyone you entrust your four-legged family member to, make sure there is a connection between the person and your pet. Make sure you are comfortable with the energy coming from them since the masseuse's energy will be transferred to your pet.

Do-It-Yourself Massage Techniques and Guidelines

NOTE: Never massage an animal that has a fever or is exhibiting signs of shock, heat stroke or distress. In these cases, get your pet to the vet! Massage is designed to increase circulation and could work against the body's natural defenses. Also if a pet has osteoporosis (fragile bones), massage could be too intense. Steer clear of areas that are bruised, blistered or show signs of a rash. For any of these conditions, talk with your Veterinarian.

1) Familiarize yourself with the basic techniques of massage:
   - **Effleurage** – Long gentle strokes in the direction of the fur using your whole flat palm and fingers.
   - **Finger Tip Pressure/Friction Massage** – Use two or three fingers or your thumbs across the muscle fibers following down the fur line in circular movements with a little shaking (but don't take your fingers off your pet's skin). Fast and invigorating, apply firm pressure but do not press deeply into muscle or tissue.

- **TTouchesTM®** – Small circular movements of the fingers and hands all over the body making one and one-quarter circles (Visualize small clock faces and go from six o'clock all the way around past six and up to nine o'clock with your fingertips). Learn more at www.ttouch.com
- **Acupressure Pointwork** – Press down gently and hold for five to thirty seconds in areas next to or between muscles, bones, vertebrae and around joints. Do not press on bony prominences or into the belly of the muscle. Exhale as you press and then inhale as you let up off the point.
- **Petrissage** – Deeper massage consisting of gentle kneading, compressing, rolling and wringing of the skin, picking up and squeezing warm, relaxed muscles.
- **Stretches** – Only after muscles have been warmed up, slowly stretch your pet's legs in their normal direction, never going past the point of resistance.
- **Tapotement** – Gentle tapping to stimulate circulation.
- **Closure** – Effleurage and then just passive touch by placing your hands for short periods of time on your pet's body without any pressure or movement.

2) Make sure your pet is ready! He shouldn't be hungry, but it is best if he hasn't eaten for at least an hour before receiving a massage. A walk or litterbox is a good idea beforehand to empty his bladder and expend energy so that he will be more willing to relax.

3) Wash your hands and then rub them together to get your energy and circulation flowing.

4) Always ask the animal for his permission before you begin. The response should be obvious, if you tune in, and you should always honor it.

5) A positive attitude is crucial! Your energy is going to be passed on to your pet, so never begin a massage if you are in a bad mood, stressed, tired or carrying negative energy of any type. Close your eyes, take a deep breath and exhale, sending your worries away while you too relax during this special time with your pooch. Try to match the cadence of your breathing to your pet's respiration so that the two of you are more in tune.

6) Create a calm ambiance by finding a quiet space. Lay a sheet on the floor, dim the lights and play soothing music at a low volume to mask distracting noises.

7) Always keep both hands on your pet throughout the massage so that you maintain a constant connection, paying attention to any feedback he gives you.

8) Be conscious of trigger points which will feel like a knot in the center of a muscle. These spots are tender, so apply light pressure with your thumb until you feel the muscle release. Then use long strokes to drain the muscle of the lactic acid.

9) Make sure you massage both sides of your pet for balance.

10) After the massage, offer your pet fresh water to help flush out the toxins and lactic acid that you have moved around. A nice walk is great but an opportunity to empty his bladder is a must before he settles into a nap dreaming of his next massage.

Other Disciplines that Aid Injuries and Promote Health in Dogs

A combination of non-invasive modalities can be used after surgery and along with massage during the course of rehabilitation therapy.

Acupuncture: Using acupuncture needles can stimulate specific points on the body resulting in various physiological effects including increased blood flow, the release of endorphins (natural pain killers), the production of cortisol which acts as an anti-inflammatory, and an increase of white blood cells and antibodies which stimulate the immune system. Besides needle insertion, acupuncture encompasses the following techniques:

- Acupressure: Administration of pressure to specific points on the body to create an effect similar to needle insertion. This is great for harder to insert locations and dogs who may not take to needles.
- Aquapuncture: Liquids (homepathics, diluted vitamins such as B12 and certain medications) are injected exerting an energetic change by pushing tissue out of their way.
- Moxibustion: Applying a heated herbal compound to needles prior to insertion. This can benefit older dogs and those suffering from joint and muscular conditions.
- Laser: A needle-less treatment for patients that don't tolerate needle insertion – a cool laser stimulates acupressure points without burning the skin or hair. See more below.
- Electrostimulation or Estim: Coursing electric current into the body between needles that have been inserted into acupuncture points can relax spasming muscles and assist the body in reestablishing nervous system impulses when nerve damage has occurred, such as spinal cord damage from a ruptured disc.

Animal Communication: Humans who possess the gift of being able to really tune into our animals may help you find out why your dog is behaving a certain way, what may ail them or any other story they wish you would know. Communicators use various techniques to do telepathic reads (like a conversation), energy dowsing (to find blocks in energy pathways), chakra scans and flower essence reads (checking for emotional balance) along with other tools to help you better know what your pet can't tell you, or you can't understand. Discovering an area of discomfort in your pet through communication could help a medical practitioner zero in on a problem and hopefully come up with a solution.

Aromatherapy: Aromatherapy is the therapeutic inhalation and topical application of pure essential oils to restore or enhance health and well-being of dogs and people. Essential oils come from various parts of aromatic plants -- the rind, flower, bark, root, resin or leaf -- that are released via steam distillation, cold expression or solvent extraction. They should not be confused with fragrance oils and potpourri, which can contain synthetic ingredients that can cause problems, such as headaches, agitation or allergic reactions. Since dogs respond well to scent and touch, calming sprays and grooming products containing pure essential oils work well when applied by hand, and at the same time can create a bonding experience for you and your pet. This "healing by scent" can comfort dogs that are anxious during storms, fireworks, travel, bath time or even veterinary visits.

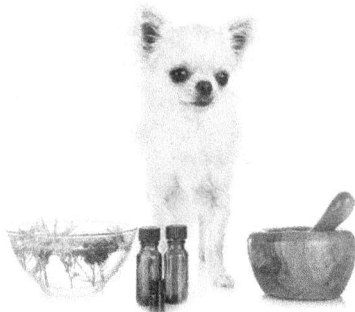

According to Vicki Rae Thorne of Earth Heart Inc., "Essential oils such as lavender, tangerine and rose geranium can have a calming effect. Bergamot has been used for anxiety, and ginger for stomach upset. Plants historically used for respiratory and immune system health include frankincense, niaouli, ravensara, lemon and thyme." It is important to work with an expert in essential oils when using them around pets. Some pets, especially cats, can have an adverse reaction to essential oils, while others can benefit greatly. The purity and quality of essential oils makes a difference. Work with a professional and understand how to use them safely around any and all of your household pets.

Chiropractic: Chiropractic manipulations or adjustments aid joints and help relax muscles by restoring misaligned vertebrae to their proper position in your dog's spinal cord. The underlying philosophy is that disease results from a disruption of nerve function, primarily caused by displaced vertebrae. When a veterinary chiropractic procedure is done, the goal is to re-align the spine relieving pressure on nerves. Followed by massage, chiropractic can be very effective.

Veterinary Orthopedic Manipulation (VOM): Not quite chiropractic, but a close cousin, Veterinary Orthopedic Manipulation (VOM) was developed by a veterinary neurologist (Dr. William Inman) who discontinued his surgical practice after seeing the outstanding benefits of this technology. VOM is a healing technique focused on returning an animal's nervous system to a healthy state. This is done with a hand held device called an Activator which reduces subluxations – misalignments of the bones. Out of place discs and joints slightly out of their socket are prime contenders for this treatment, and problems may be found with this method months prior to them showing up on x-rays. Most pets tolerate the light pressure and if repeated, the process actually releases endorphins causing the animal to relax. When fired down the spine, the Activator can open up blockages in the nerve bundles on either side aiding the various internal organs as well.

Hydrotherapy/Underwater Treadmill: The buoyancy of water allows exercise with less stress to the joints and can have cardiovascular benefits. The warmth of the water helps increase circulation, relax muscles and allows for greater flexibility and range of motion. Hydrotherapy can also decrease inflammation and swelling and reduce pain levels.

Hyperbaric Oxygen Therapy (HBOT): Hyperbaric comes from the Greek word "hyper" meaning "more" and "baric" relating to pressure. A hyperbaric oxygen chamber increases the pressure allowing a patient's body to absorb much larger quantities of oxygen than it would if it was not under pressure. When oxygen is inhaled at normal atmospheric pressure, it is transported on hemoglobin in the red blood cells. Under pressure, however, oxygen dissolves in the plasma, cerebrospinal fluid in the brain and spinal cord, lymph and other body fluids making it more easily delivered to the tissues, including those with poor blood supply.

Oxygen deprivation due to poor circulation, injury, surgery and other causes can hinder healing and impair function, which is why HBOT benefits so many diverse conditions including:

- Snakebites and Traumatic Injuries such as crushing, swelling & major vessel tears
- Pressure Sores & Chronic Wounds
- Carbon Monoxide Poisoning
- Severe Anemia
- Severe Gastrointestinal Illness
- Bone Infections
- Stroke

One of the most dramatic examples of oxygen deprivation would be during a stroke. A blockage or bleeding in the brain's blood vessels disrupts the flow of oxygen as well as nutrient-rich blood. Cells in the affected area die or are damaged, but when these areas are infused with massive amounts of oxygen during a hyperbaric oxygen treatment, damaged brain cells may literally wake up.

LLLT/Cold Laser/Therapeutic Laser: Low-Level Laser Therapy, Low Level Light Therapy or "cold laser" is a non-thermal light energy used to stimulate healing, reduce inflammation and provide pain relief. Benefits may include stimulation of both cartilage and collagen and can assist dogs suffering from arthritis, tendonitis, muscle spasm and various wounds.

Nutrition: Proper nutrients are critical to create a healthy immune system and good body condition. Proper nutrition can add several years to your dog's life and delay the need for medication for chronic diseases such as osteoarthritis. You may want to consider supplements depending on the nutrition path that you've chosen for your dogs as no one diet is perfect for every dog. Speak with a professional to customize what may help your animal thrive. See pages 14-18 for more nutrition information.

Holistic Approach: Increasingly, pet parents are considering alternative treatments for their pets for a variety of reasons. A holistic approach is one that factors in the entire body and being of the pet – it looks at the big picture and sees how everything is working together to create a whole and healthy animal. Rather than fixing a problem, it seeks the root causes addressing it in a "gentle healing" method for long-term results. More and more Veterinarians and other professionals are incorporating holistic and homeopathic treatments and approaches into western medicine. If this is something that resonates with you, seek out a specialized professional in that area and discuss the options and expectations.

Knowledge is power and more and more is discovered each year in our quest to help dogs live longer, happier, healthier lives. Take advantage of the seminars and workshops, webinars, websites, good old fashioned books and the expertise of professionals who live to help pets thrive.

Refer to the charts and forms in the back of this book and be proactive by filling them out and seeking out the information you don't currently possess.

You are your dog's advocate and protector.

Notes: _____

_____

_____

_____

_____

_____

_____

_____

_____

_____

CBD for your Dogs

CBD has been gaining in popularity in the pet world as way to address a variety of wide ranging health and wellness conditions. Though research on it and the Endocannabinoid System (ECS) are still in what would deemed the early stages, compared to other body systems, there is much to be encouraged by from what has been researched, as well as a multitude of anecdotal evidence.

So What is CBD?
CBD is an acronym for Cannabidiol (Can-a-bid-i-ol), a naturally occurring class of molecules called cannabinoids abundant in the plant genus Cannabis Sativa L. CBD makes up close to 40% of the plant and is just one of over 100 cannabinoids presently identified in cannabis sativa. CBD interacts with an animal's naturally occurring endocannabinoid system, and is non-psychoactive because there is little to no THC (tetrahydrocannabinol). In brief, CBD or PCR (Phyto Cannabinoid Rich) sativa plants having low levels of THC are referred to as Hemp and Marijuana plants are those with high levels of THC.

A bit more about Hemp vs. Marijuana Hemp and marijuana are related, but the differences can be night and day.

- First off, the plants look different. One of the oldest domestic crops grown, tall, sturdy hemp plants were farmed by early civilizations for food, oil, shelter and textiles. Similar to bamboo, shoots can grow 15 feet high. Marijuana plants however, tend to grow as low and bushy.
- As far as cultivation, hemp is grown for its stalks and seeds and marijuana for its leaves and flowers.
- The elevated levels of THC in marijuana are responsible for its signature "high," while hemp has very little THC. A study done by a private laboratory in Denver (Charas Scientifi c) found that recreational marijuana contains up to 30% THC while the hemp used to create products for pets and people contains a maximum legal amount of .03%. Some companies even go through a costly process to remove all traces of THC in hemp products to improve safety.
- Both hemp and marijuana contain CBD, but the hemp plant produces more, making it the preferred choice to battle anxiety, chronic pain, epilepsy and other ailments. Since CBD does not cause a "high," it is considered a holistic treatment, not a pharmaceutical one.

So keep in mind that CBD and Marijuana are definitely not the same and only one – CBD – is safe for pets. Never ever share edibles, THC or any human-specific cannabis products with your dog! "The number-one animal ER issue in states in which medical and/or recreational marijuana is legal is marijuana intoxication," says Dr. Robin Downing, DVM and a pain medicine veterinary specialist

Are all CBD oils created equal?

No. Many CBD oils on the market are NOT naturally occurring NOR are they truly full spectrum CBD. Most undergo a form of chemical synthesis that requires lab manipulation - compounds are taken out during the extraction process and synthesized ones added in. In order to be considered a truly full spectrum CBD oil (which is what you want for your pet), it should contain naturally occurring (Phyto-Cannabinoid Rich) therapeutic parts of the plant. You need to know how the plants were grown and how the compounds were extracted in order to get the best quality CBD oil for your dog!

The hemp plant is considered a hyper-accumulator which means it readily absorbs anything in the soil. So it is even important to know what kinds of soil, and what pest control methods were used in the growth of the plants.

How does it work?

Dogs, cat, humans, all invertebrates (except insects) have an endocannabinoid system that helps maintain the physiological, neurological and immunological systems of the body -- it modulates our emotions, response to pain and other sensations. If there is a deficiency anywhere, multiple receptors can use CBD oil to help the body get into balance or achieve homeostasis. We still have much to learn yet findings are already showing the symbiotic relationship between the Endocannabinoid system in our bodies and CBD.

A wonderful benefit of how CBD interacts with the body's own endocannabinoid system is known as the entourage effect. This is when the many components within the cannabis plant interact with the body to produce a stronger influence than any one of those components alone. When we combine multiple compounds, we don't end up with the sum of each part but exponentially increase their effects.

How much CBD oil should I give my dog?

CBD interacts with your pet's endocannabinoid system, which means their reaction is dependent on their tolerance as well as immunity. In other words, every dog is a bit different. Surprisingly, CBD dosage is not dependent exclusively on weight, however it can be a guideline. "Start low and go slow" until you achieve the results you are seeking for your dog is the mantra. Recommend basic dosage - with a minimum to strong dosage range - is suggested between 1-5 mg. for every 10 pounds of weight.

While there is more to learn about CBD (AKA – PCR Hemp Oil), it is showing to be a multi-modality aid for pain, nausea, anxiety and a number of other ailments without causing the organ and tissue damage NSAIDs (anti-inflammatory meds), anti-convulsants and other pharmaceuticals can cause.

READING YOUR DOG'S BODY LANGUAGE

On a daily basis, study your dog and learn to communicate with him, gaining his trust and paying close attention to what he is trying to say through Body Language. When any animal is upset or not feeling well, even your own best friend, they might be grumpy and could nip, so it's important to stay alert to changes in their ears, eyes, tail, vocalization and muscle tension. Any animal (just like a human) may be in a good mood one moment and then do a 180, so stay alert to even the slightest changes.

The following is a general guideline but knowing your own dog's personality is the best measure. Additional drawings are in the Resource Section of this book to get you better acquainted as to what the various behaviors look like.

	Happy Dog	Grumpy Pup	Frightened Fido	Sick Dog
Ears	Flat	Flat & Pressed Back Against Head	Pulled Back Against Head	To The Sides Or Any Abnormal Position
Eyes	Open & Bright	Pupils Narrow	Wide Open	Half Crossed
Hackles (Fur on the neck back)	Relaxed & Smooth Fur	Fluffed Up	Fluffed Up	Could Go Either Way
Tails	Relaxed or upright especially if the tip of the tail is curled can mean "howdy" from a dog. May lower front legs with butt in the air waggin tail with a "play bow"	Swishing with hair bristled or straight up like a bottle brush; dogs may still be wagging so beware.	Tucked between legs or he'll bow with hair standing straight up.	Tucked Between Legs
Sounds	Happy bark that sounds like "Play With Me" from dogs	Low gutteral sounds or growls from dogs	Frightened cry to growing	

Proper Handling

When just holding a puppy or small dog, it is best to make them feel secure by holding their body against yours with one hand supporting the hind quarters (don't let legs dangle stretching their back in an awkward position) and the other hand behind the front legs supporting the chest.

Small dogs, can be swaddled in a towel to further restrain them and prevent nails from scratching you while performing observations or doing various procedures. Restrain means "to hold back or suppress," so sometimes we restrain a pet to protect ourselves (muzzling for instance) and other times to prevent them from danger. Leashes, collars, harnesses, carriers, crates and dog runs, even our own two hands, are all forms of restraint to keep a pet out of harm's way. In serious situations and under veterinary care, anesthesia or sedation would be used as a form of restraint to allow professionals to tend to your dog with safety in mind for themselves and the dog.

To learn more about muzzling and restraining for at-home procedures, turn to page 110 in the Dog First-Aid section of this book.

INTRODUCTIONS

Introducing Your Dog to a New Canine Family Member:

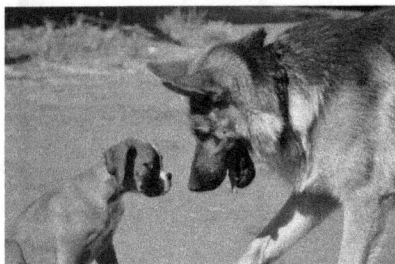

Neutral turf is rule number one! If the shelter or location you are adopting from will allow you to bring your current dog there to meet your prospective new one, it is a good idea so you can see how it will work before you officially adopt. Even allowing the two dogs to sniff towels/blankets the other has slept on can be a good first step.

For the first meeting you will need a second person so that each of you can handle one dog on-leash. Let them casually walk back and forth without letting them pay the other much attention. When that is going well (no pulling or lunging), bring the dogs together and walk both together side-by-side but avoiding contact. Make both sit while the humans talk, then walk away. On the next pass, let the two dogs sniff and greet each other (still on-leash). If all is going well and you are in a secured fence, drop the leashes and let them play but do not take your eyes off the dogs and be prepared to grab leashes. "Wiggly" and relaxed body posture is good. Immediately break up any staring which could result in a quarrel.

When it's time for them both to come home, have them enter the yard first if at all possible and then enter the house together.

Make sure there are doubles of everything so that there is no need for competition – double water and food bowls, bedding, toys, etc. If either dog is known to be possessive or have resource guarding instincts, remove toys for the initial few weeks. It's a good idea to keep food and water bowls at a distance from each other and show the new dog where his things are located.

It is best to bring a new pet home when you have several days to stay home with both pets and get them acclimated to their new situation -- a weekend or when you can take a few days off. Like with human kids, take care not to show preferences, but do treat or pet your previous dog first until they work out who the alpha dog (leader of the pack) is.

Mostly, dogs and cats like stability -- a routine -- so any environmental or social change may have a pronounced effect on their behavior. You may find your well-mannered pooch soiling the carpet or chewing up your bed spread once a new dog joins the family. Be patient. Show them both plenty of love and affection. Animals are adaptable, but it may take time, and every animal is different. Don't throw your hands up in distress after only a few weeks. Patience and TLC will see you through and your reward will be double the unconditional love.

A change in behavior without an obvious change in situation, however, could be a health concern. Your Veterinarian may suggest an animal behaviorist to get to the root of the issue.

Introducing Dogs to Cats

Some do fine. Some cannot live safely together. The first rule is proceed cautiously during introductions having at least two people present, one ready to intervene with each animal if need be.

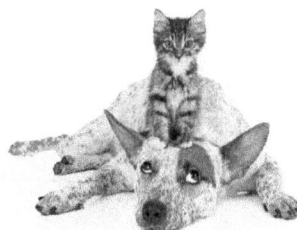

Keep the dog on a loose lead and observe his body language at all times. The other person should pay attention to the cat's reactions. Do not push the animals together. If the cat is not raising her hackles (the fur on her back) or hissing, allow her to move freely around the room. If the dog is not acting aggressively, praise him as he allows the cat to move around, even sniffing the dog if she wishes.Dogs with strong prey instincts will become focused, staring, stiffening, whining and/ or barking. If these behaviors are present or if the dog lunges, calmly put the cat in another room with a tall baby gate while one person distracts the dog playing with a toy.

When set up with the cat in another room with all her supplies and a tall and sturdy baby gate installed in the door, allow the dog periodic loose leash visits to see the cat on the other side of the gate. Once the cat no longer creates such a rise in the dog, sit comfortably on the floor on the dog's side of the gate and reach through, petting the cat and feeding her treats on her side while you do the same with the dog.

Your goal is to lessen your dog's interest in your feline companion, but in some cases, instinct is strong and the two may never be left safely alone. If introductions are not going well, seek a professional behaviorist. In the worst circumstances, a dog can quickly injure or kill a cat and cats can inflict devastating eye injuries on dogs. Calm, patient baby steps are the best route to getting these two species comfortable around each other.

Introducing your Dog to Your New Baby

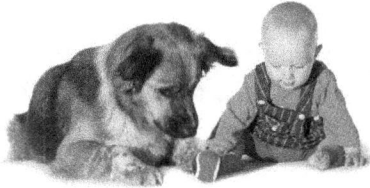

Dogs, like their two-legged counterparts, can cope with big changes in their lives if we take the time to help them through. A new human brother or sister joining the family is an exciting time for all but can be stressful with added noise, stressed out parents and possibly less time for belly rubs and walks in the park. Doing your homework and properly preparing your dog can make for a smooth transition. Don't wait for the day your newborn comes home to start telling your fur child how to behave! You are setting him up for disaster if you do so and that is completely unfair.

If you haven't already, start looking at your dog like you are his parent too. Is he lacking manners and socialization that could prove dangerous around a baby or even pregnant you? It may be fun when your dog drags you down the stairs and out the door anxious for his walk or jumps up with paws on your shoulder. These habits though won't be fun during your second and third trimester. Start now correcting any behaviors you've, up to now, over looked. Gently tug, bump and squeeze his paws a little at a time to accustom him to how the baby might touch him. If he responds well, praise, praise, praise! If he is uncomfortable, he needs to learn to walk away to his own space and not snap or growl. If your dog won't let you get away with this "tougher" handling, he or she certainly won't let the baby.

A big change for your dog with the baby's arrival will be the amount of time you get to devote to him each day. Do not ignore him, but start preparing him by varying meal and walk times and quality versus quantity of special time together. Make sure he has a special space to retreat to and plenty of toys to keep him busy when you can't. Begin weaning your pet off dog toys that in any way resemble baby toys. Find play things for Fido that are uniquely different so that there won't be confusion later on with your dog thinking the baby has his toy!

Do let your dog explore the nursery as you set it up and accustom him to the movements of an empty stroller. Even practice with a doll in the stroller going for walks together. Can you picture your first walk with dog on a leash pulling you down the street or getting entangled in the stroller wheels with the baby along for the ride? Let people ooh and ahh over the doll so that your dog can get used to the attention a real baby will be getting. If you have friends with babies, having them visit and letting your dog meet their babies under supervision can be a great help. Always let the pet go slowly to the baby. Do not push a baby into an animal's face! Practice helps smooth the way and helps your pet learn what to expect.

Practicing with the car seat, travel barrier and/or crate is a must! Practice with your dog before the baby arrives so that he knows there is still a place for him too. If you haven't practiced proper safety with your dog carefully in a dog seat belt, now is the time to start. Get him used to his restraint and a doll in the car seat as well. If the doll doesn't make noise, ask friends who have a baby to make a few recordings you can play for your dog while he rides, when he's napping and even at meal time. When he responds appropriately praise and treat him. Help them learn to adjust to the new sounds and smells. Let them sniff baby powders and oils on your hands, baby wipes and even the smell of pureed carrots long before baby comes home.

While you are in the hospital, a great trick is to send home a blanket or clothing the baby has slept on or worn. Then let your dog get familiar with the scent before the baby's homecoming.

When the moment arrives for introductions, come in first without the baby so your dog can give you their proper greeting and you'll have free hands to return their affection. Once the initial hellos have been accomplished, have another family member bring in the baby and slowly let your pooch meet his new "brother or sister." Watch body language but remember...pets pick up your vibes, so stay calm but alert. Take care with your voice. "Baby talk" to your baby could be mistaken for the sounds you use for your pup and might sound like an invitation for him to play or interact with the baby.

Although baby will be foremost on your mind, try to give your dog as much one-on-one time as possible. Don't ship him off to "boarding school," but maybe an occasional day at doggie day care will give Fido a break as well as you. Having spent time teaching him his down/stay commands and playing quietly with toys in his special space will really pay off now.

No matter how well things are going, NEVER EVER leave your baby and dog alone together...little dog or big dog. An animal's natural instincts could be triggered by a crying or cooing infant.

Whether you share your life with a puppy or a mature dog, remember too that you will be bringing all types of new things into the house and many may drop and land on the floor. Pay due diligence to keep your dog safe from pins, buttons and anything that your pup could swallow or could cause him harm.

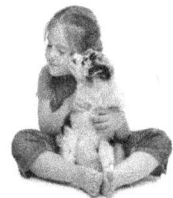

A dog should never lose his home when a human comes in to the world. Plan ahead for a happy lifetime together.

Show patience and love, always supervise and stay alert to your dog's and your baby's changing attitudes so you can quickly make any corrections along the way. Think about little things like keeping your dogs well-groomed and practice training to be sure they continue to mind their manners. If things aren't going well, don't delay. Seek the immediate help of a professional behaviorist or trainer to nip it in the bud. With love, patience and effort, you can enjoy watching your child and dog becoming loyal companions and playmates.

On a final note, keep in mind the amazing ways your dog will HELP with your baby:

- Baby Monitor: Dogs and their amazing ears will be on high alert.

- Entertainment: Giggles and smiles will ensue when baby watches puppy play.

- Immune Booster: Studies have shown that the exposure to germs from dogs challenges a child's immune system leading to fewer respiratory illnesses and ear infections as well as a decreased risk for asthma and allergies later in life.

- Exercise: Your pooch will remind you it's time to get up and moving, so that the three of you can get fresh air and sunshine on two-feet, four-paws or stroller wheels.

- Clean-up: Who needs a plastic mat under the high chair when Fido is ready, willing and able to do clean-up? Just make sure what drops is canine safe and that they do not take food from the child.

- Unconditional Love: There's nothing a child needs in never-ending supply more than love and your happy, well-mannered dog is a perfect source of unwavering devotion.

Be sure to read about "Zooeyia" on page 6 to understand more fully the benefits our four-legged friends can have on your child and on you.

Introducing your Dog to Visitors/Strangers

Having your dog meet family and friends can be an exciting and rewarding time. Particularly if the people are not pet savvy, talk to them ahead about what to expect and what you'd prefer they do and don't do when Fido greets them. Sudden movements, hand clapping and foot stomping can scare or put your pooch on guard. Also beware that although some people may say, "I love animals," they could be referring to the older fluffy Maltese they had as a child and not your rambunctious two-year old Labrador who thinks he's a lap dog, so give them a heads-up as to your dog's personality so that everyone starts off on the right paw. Having a brief phone conversation with visitors prior to their ringing the bell will help keep the peace. Remind them to pull closed screen doors and latch any gates, not to feed your dog unless you provide a treat and to watch what they bring into your home (medication in purses, cigarettes and lighters). Also advise them not to wear hoods, hats or sun glasses as many dogs go ballistic at the way these items change the human shape.

As the person enters, have your dog stay away from the door, but let them know when it's okay to nose over. After your pup has had a good sniff, tell the person to offer the back of their hand for an additional nose-over and then to gently extend their fingers under the dog's chin for a gentle scratching or petting. Children in particular must learn not to pat a dog on the head which looks like a slap or hit to the dog and can immediately make him defensive.

It's often a good idea if you have a treat outside the door waiting for your visitor to offer to your pet at this point. Should your dog jump up on the person, have them turn their back and remain quiet until the dog sits or stops the action. "Off" and "Leave It" are commands often taught to stop jumping.

Some dogs do quite well when strangers are sitting, but bark at them every time your company stands or moves about. This is a territorial and guarding issue and also the dog is just not sure what the person's intent is. Often with continued visits, your pet becomes more relaxed and that brings up an important socialization issue: if you do want visitors at your home, start early on with your dog so that they become accustomed. If they've lived with you for years before another person ever comes over, it could make life difficult when even the cable guy or refrigerator repairman pays a visit.

Dog Friendly Kid Tips

To safely share our lives with our four-legged friends, there are **Grrreat tips every human should follow,** no matter their number of years on the planet:

Never, ever leave a child alone with a pet!!!

NEVER

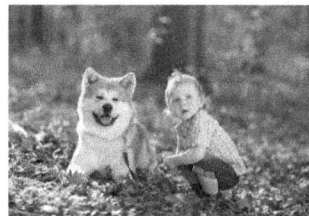

- Tease animals by pulling their ears or tails.
- Throw things at them, ride or chase them.
- Go near tied up or chained animals.
- Touch or play with an animal while he is eating or sleeping.
- Steal toys or bones.
- Run or scream if an animal comes near you and never run towards him.
- Stare into an animal's eyes.
- Do not pat him on the head. This looks like you are going to hit him. Instead, let him sniff the back of your hand (after you have asked permission to pet the animal) and if the pet seems agreeable, extend your fingers and slowly beginning to scratch under his chin and neck.

ALWAYS

- Act kindly and gently towards animals.
- Ask if it is okay before you pet a dog. Respect that some dogs may be working on the job as in guide dogs and therapy dogs, but even if a family pet, it is always polite and smart to ask first!
- Stand still like a tree if an animal comes near you, and allow him to sniff you first. Then scratch under his chin if he seems agreeable, but never raise your hand above his head which looks like a slap.
- Lie face down like a log and cover the back of your neck if you are attacked by an animal.
- Tell an adult if you see a stray or injured animal.

Animals can magically put a smile on any human face. For all they do for us, we must learn to treat them with compassion and learn to speak their language, allowing them their own space and time.

BASIC DOG CARE

Seven "DOG GONE GOOD TO KNOW" Rules to Help YOU Help YOUR Dog

1) Give your pets a weekly *Head-to-Tail Check-up* monitoring respiration, pulse, capillary refill time and feeling for lumps & bumps, fleas, ticks, foxtails, etc. Finding a lump early and getting it checked could save your pet's life. Observe your dog's normal habits (notice how much he drinks, eats, urinates & defecates); notice his stance and how he sits. If you know what's normal for your pet, you can quickly notice something that is not and alert your Veterinarian. (See page 232)

2) Spay or Neuter your dog and take him to the Veterinarian for *annual check-ups*, including wellness or geriatric testing once your pet reaches age 7. Keep good records on your dog's health, licensing and care issues, and learn where your closest animal emergency center is in case your vet is closed when you need him.

3) Always have *ID tags* on your dog and get them micro-chipped so that others can help them find their way home should they ever become separated from you. Keep these identifiers up-to-date and make sure tags are legible as they tend to become difficult to read after rubbing against other tags on your dog's collar.

4) *Socialize & Obedience Train & Exercise your dog.*
A well-trained dog is less likely to get into trouble and a well-socialized canine will become a more-welcomed member of the family. *Always keep your dog on a leash or in a fenced yard* so that you can keep him safe from traffic (the #1 most preventable injury to dogs and man), other animals, pesticides that might be on your neighbor's lawn, poisons in garbage cans and more. Many well-meaning owners expose their pets to needless dangers by allowing their animals to run loose. Since we've domesticated the canine, changed their landscape and created motor cars and super highways, we have an obligation to restrict our Dogs' boundaries to keep them out of harm's way. How often have you seen a dog or cat hit by a car on a street near you? You certainly don't want your four-legged friend to suffer this fate. Additionally, stray pets are often killed by other animals, poisoned, contract disease or are sold to labs for experimentation. Regardless of the size of land you inhabit, it is imperative that you create a big enough world at home for your animals to explore and thrive in.

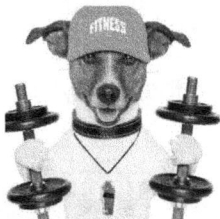

Exercise your pet. Keep your pet's body and mind stimulated for a long, happy and healthy life. Boredom is the playground for bad habits and destructive behaviors. Digging can lead to Houdini-like escapes landing your loving canine in a shelter or hit by a car while injuries can be caused from items torn, ingested or broken. Physical activity and fresh air does a canine body good, but so does time spent with you!

5) Feed a *high quality, age-appropriate food* (puppy food for puppies, senior food for older dogs, light food for overweight pups) and read those labels so that you know what you're really feeding your dog. Also give supplements for long-term nutritional therapy which protect your pet from the inside out & provide nutrients commercial food may lack. Check with your Veterinarian or pet nutritionist to find out what is advised.

6) Finally, please make sure you keep your pet's body & mind stimulated with plenty of fresh air, *exercise and time spent with YOU.*

7. *Know Dog Safety & Learn Dog First Aid & CPCR* (see Section Two)…It could save a life! Also put together a *Dog First-Aid Kit* (page 111) so that you'll have the tools to do the job.

Weekly Head-to-Tail Check-up (also see page 232)

Really get to know your dog and you'll more quickly identify something 'not quite right!' Getting your pooch used to your touch not only can help you find a small problem before it becomes a nightmare, but will also make your pet's Health & Safety Team happier since they (your Veterinarian, groomer and pet sitter) will find him much easier to handle. Keep a record of your observations on the diagram located in the resource section of this book entitled "Head To Tail". (See page 232)

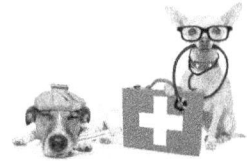

Look & feel your dog over from head-to-tail:

- Check ears for foul odor or redness.
- Make sure eyes look clear, pupils are equally dilated and there's no excessive tearing.
- Doggy breath should not be offensive; smelling sweet or like nail polish remover could signal kidney problems.
- Feel for lumps and bumps - catching a tumor early could save a life.
- If your dog's skin is flaky or his coat is dull, bathe, brush and add Omega 3s to his diet.
- Remove parasites, burrs or foxtails.
- Check paw pads for cracks and make sure nails are trimmed short.
- Keep private areas clean.

Notice changes in your dog's behavior or routine. If your dog is requiring you to perform these tasks more or less frequently he may need a check-up:

- Refilling water bowls
- Amount of food being consumed
- How often he asks to go outside
- Soiled spots in the house

Get familiar with what your pet looks like when he sits, stands and walks.
"Yes" to any of these questions means it's time for a visit to your Veterinarian:

- Is his posture unusual?
- Is it more difficult for my pet to get up or lie down or does he moan when doing so?
- Is he leaning to one side or favoring a limb?
- Is he less active?

Check	Your Dog Is Good To Go	How You Can Help	Your Dog Needs To Go To The Veterinarian
Ears	Pink and Smell Good	Wax debris - clean with ear wash	Foul odor, redness or ear mites which look like coffee grounds
Eyes	Bright & clear, pupils are equally dilated & responsive; no excessive tearing	Excessive Tearing - Flush with saline solution or eye wash	Cloudiness to eyes; one pupil larger than the other; excessive tearing not alleviated by saline solution or eye wash; squinting or pawing at eye.
Nose	Shiny & Moist		Dry & cracked excessively dripping; mucus discharge; sneezing; open wound.
Mouth	Clean white teeth with no bad odor; scissor bite from teeth meeting properly; pink moist gums with CRTs 2 seconds	Brush daily with pet specific toothpaste. Keep dog well hydrated.	Foul odor, tartar build up; redness obvious absess or loose teeth; uneven bite; brightened, blue, pale or white; dry or tacky gums.
Skin & Coat	Shiny, no lumps, or bumps or flakes; healthy pink; no hair loss.	Bathe, brush regularly & add Omega 3s to your dog's diet.	Lumps, bumps, scabs, open sores; bald spots or extreme hair loss.
Legs & Paws	When walking, gait is smooth & even. No cuts to pads; nails short; dog stands and moves well with no tenderness.	Clean any pads wounds. Don't let them walk on hot or extremely cold surfaces; trim nails ; exercise.	Open wounds; limping; unsteadiness; difficulty walking;, getting up or lying down; dragging a limb.
Chest & Abdomen	Pink skin, no lumps, bumps or tender areas.; you can feel ribs but not see them and chest is lower than the tummy	Keep your dog at a healthy weight.	Any lumps or tenderness; need to lose excessive weight.
Heart	Steady even rythm. 60 - 160 Beats Per Minute for Medium to Large Dogs 90-220 Beats Pet Minute for small dogs and cats	Get regular veterinary check ups and appropriate exercise.	Murmur or uneven heart beats (arrhythmia); faster or slower rate of BPM than normal.

Check	Your Dog Is Good To Go	How You Can Help	Your Dog Needs To Go To The Veterinarian
Lungs	Clear inhalation and exhalation. 10 - 30 Beats Per Minute for Medium to Large Dogs 20 - 40 Beats Pet Minute for small dogs	Get regular veterinary check ups and appropriate exercise.	Labored or difficult breathing; raspy; muffled, congested; rate higher or lower than normal.
Privates	Clean, No discharge, normal size.	If pet can't reach, clean with soft, warm damp cloth	Red, unusual discharge; swollen
Tail	Shiny coat , no lumps, or bumps		Hair loss, open sores, lumps/bumps
Habits	Good energy level and appetitie; doesn't drink water excessively; regular bathroom habits	Feed high quality and age appropriate food; provide fresh, clean water and proper exercise.	Lethargic; loss or increase of appetite / thirst. Change in bathroom habits - more or less frequent "accidents", vomit or diarrhea.

Dental Care – A Clean Mouth Can Mean a Healthy Dog

Brush your dog's teeth regularly for good overall health. Bacteria in the mouth can travel through the bloodstream resulting in damage to the kidneys, heart valves and other organs.

If you notice any of these signs, it's time for a check-up:

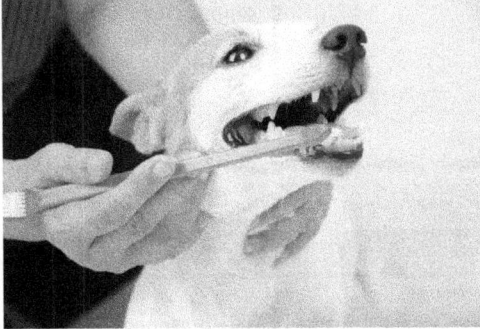

- bad breath
- loose teeth
- visible tartar (brownish-yellow stains)
- swelling under the eyes
- difficulty eating
- excessive drooling
- red, irritated, swollen or bleeding gums
- loss of appetite or weight loss
- lethargy or loss of energy

NOTE: Toothaches can make anyone grouchy and result in bad behavior! If your dog suddenly has bad manners, it could be a medical issue.

ABCs of Brushing Your Dog's Teeth:

- If your dog is not used to your fingers in his mouth, dip your finger in non-sodium, onion free chicken broth and rub his gums but don't let him nibble your fingers.
- After a few days of finger massaging, try a dog-specific toothbrush and pet tooth paste. It comes in several flavors so find which one he likes best.
- Place your hand around your dog's muzzle (you can actually keep his mouth closed), lift his lip on one side and in a circular motion, brush the outsides of the top and bottom teeth – 30 seconds on the top set, 30 seconds on the bottom and then move to the other side. If your dog is reluctant, do just a few teeth, praise him and try again the next day.

Grooming - Keeping up Appearances in Between Trips to the Groomer

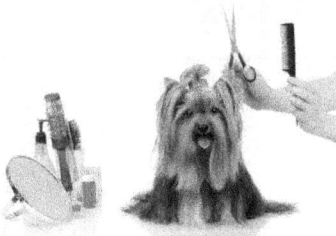

Your dog needs regular grooming because just like you, they feel better when they are clean and healthy.

Start when your puppy is young so that grooming becomes a fun thing to do together.

- First brush your dog's coat out thoroughly removing all tangles, mats and snarls. Brush in the same direction that the hair grows with a brush recommended by your groomer or pet store for his particular coat. Brush gently but everywhere -- behind ears, on his belly, tail and legs. Matted fur can cause sores as well as trap heat close to your pet's body.

- There are many types of shampoo, so read labels and don't use ones with products you can't pronounce. Natural is better, and never use a "flea dip" on your puppy, senior dog or a sick pet as they contain harsh chemicals.
- Bathe your dog in a tub of warm water and work shampoo into a good lather avoiding his eyes, nostrils and mouth. Place large cotton balls in his ears to prevent water from getting in, and be sure to rinse off all soap from your dog's skin and fur.
- Remove cotton balls and carefully wipe the insides of both ears with a soft cloth – never a cotton swab which can damage the ear canal.
- Towel dry then brush and thoroughly dry your dog's coat keeping him warm.
- Trim nails with special dog nail clippers to prevent them from getting caught in rugs, furniture and humans.

Some dogs have coats with two layers: the hair you can see, and a hidden, soft and dense layer -- Newfoundlands, Retrievers, Akitas, Shepherds and Huskies to name a few. This undercoat helps a dog stay warm and dry in cold weather and it protects from the hot sun too. so get your dog clean all under, but never shave down to the skin, as fur insulates from sunburn as well as thorns and burrs.

Nail Trimming:

First and foremost, get your dog used to having their paws played with. Touch and gently squeeze paws and look them over from day one.

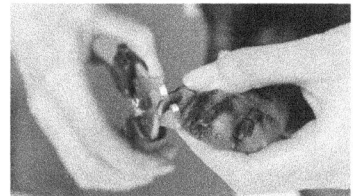

- Make sure nail clippers are sharp.
- Gently squeeze toe and place an unlit wooden match stick firmly underneath and clip only the matchstick so that your pet gets used to the sound of the clipper and the pressure applied.
- When ready (this could be an entirely separate day), clip the real thing but pay close attention to the "quick," small blood vessel that runs down the nail and will bleed considerably if cut. On white nails it is dark pink or brown and you want to clip just shy of it. On dark nails take off only a little of the nail at the time until you reach the quick.
- When you look at the cut edge of the nail, you will see a dark center known as the quick when you have cut sufficiently. Being exposed to the air for a couple weeks causes the quick to recede so you can clip again to get the nails shorter without causing bleeding, but...
  - If you cut into the quick, you will hurt your pet and will jeopardize the chance of your pet ever sitting still for a nail trim.
  - You may need to perform first-aid (see page 140) to stop the bleeding; so be prepared to help anytime you do a nail trim.

Anal Glands:

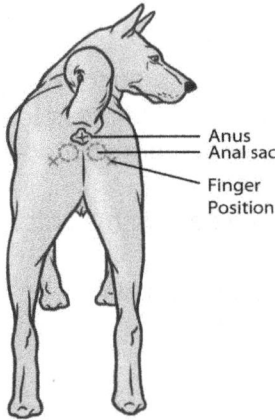

Shaped like a pea, the two anal glands are located just under the skin at the four o'clock and eight o' clock position under the tail and below the anus.

Their nasty smelling fluid is produced by dogs, cats and other small mammals to give their stool a unique scent, a way to identify the individual animal.

Groomers often express the anal glands during a bath, but if Fido has never had a problem, it may not be necessary so consult with your Veterinarian.
Learn more on page 130.

Parasites: Flea & Tick Free:

Parasites can cause itching, redness and unpleasant skin problems, so keep your pet flea and tick free with preventive treatments recommended by your Veterinarian. Insect-borne diseases can be a serious health risk to people and pets but there is controversy over the safety of applying commercial insecticides, so you may want to consider effective alternatives.

Homeopathic Tip:

- Neem seed oil, from an evergreen tree native to India, has been used as a remedy for a wide variety of skin problems. At 2-3% it is an effective insect repellent although it has a strong scent your pet may not appreciate. Unlike commercial insecticides that can indiscriminately kill insects, neem oil only affects those that chew or suck. When ingested, it disrupts the bug's normal functions making him forget to eat, fly or lay eggs resulting in a diminished population.
- Food grade diatomaceous earth also can keep fleas away from your pets. Diatomaceous earth is a fine powder made from the crushed, fossilized remains of a marine algae. When used in flea prevention, its roughness cuts the flea as it moves causing it to leak water (which the diatomaceous earth absorbs), dehydrating the flea. (You and your pets should be careful and not inhale the diatomaceous earth).

If you discover a tick:

- Slick your dog's hair away from tick and place a cotton ball soaked in rubbing alcohol on the tick. This often causes the tick to back out of your dog for easy removal.
- If that doesn't work, pull tick with tweezers, getting tips close to dog's body without pulling his hair or skin. Do not attempt to suffocate the tick with petroleum jelly or nail polish which results in the tick regurgitating his stomach contents into your pooch. Also, do not try to burn the tick with a match as you'll probably burn your dog, and do not pull a tick with your fingers. By doing so, you'll squeeze its abdomen causing it to regurgitate its stomach contents into your pet!

- Cleanse with peroxide and apply antibiotic ointment. The oxygen in 3% hydrogen Peroxide destroys Lyme disease bacteria so pour it liberally on the skin over bites on light-haired dogs (but do keep away from their eyes). For darker-furred pets, it's a good idea to apply the peroxide using an eyedropper. This way you can deliver it directly on the skin and avoid it bleaching out the richer colored fur. It is however much better to have a Lyme Disease-free pet than to worry about a patch of lighter fur. Be aware that if you suspect the tick could be a carrier, save the tick and take it and your pet to the vet for testing. Always be vigilant for signs of infection.

A tick's mouth parts penetrate your dog's skin to suck blood and can leave disease behind, so it's a good idea to keep the tick in a zip lock baggie (after drowning tick in water or alcohol – never crush the tick as that spreads bacteria) in case your dog has a reaction. Your Veterinarian can then determine type of tick and any disease it was carrying.

Know & Vaccinate Against Diseases OR... Get a Titer Test

The best protection you can give your dog from certain diseases is to provide regular vaccinations. As puppies and kittens, they receive their immunity from the colostrum in their momma's milk, but once weaned, the antibodies wane so they need injected antigens to create immunity from disease. Think of it as arming your dog's immune system with the correct weapon needed to kill off a specific disease. Research has proven that many vaccinations no longer need to be given annually as protection can last for many years, so discuss with your Veterinarian how infrequently you may safely revaccinate your dog. Humans don't get booster shots annually – actually, many of the vaccinations we receive as children keep us immune for our lifetime, so it's no wonder that dogs, may also not need frequent injections. Too much of a good thing may not be good for your pet when over-vaccination has possible adverse effects (tumors at the sight of the injection, neurological or kidney issues to name a few).

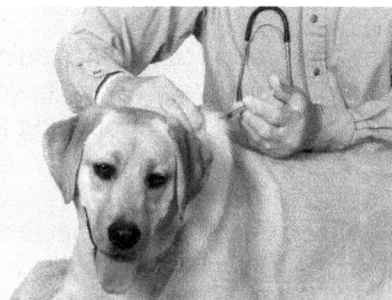

When your dog is due for a booster, discuss titer testing with your Veterinarian. A titer test is a blood sample that when observed on a slide, can determine the level of your dog's immunity to a specific disease. It measures the immune system's preparedness to fight infection and is actually the only proof that your dog has created the antibodies needed to protect itself. Approximately 1 out of every 1,000 pets are non-responders. This means their bodies do not react to the vaccination and fail to create protective antibodies, so getting a vaccination doesn't guarantee that your pet will avoid illness.

In the past titer testing was generally more costly than getting a vaccination, however new technologies are making it more convenient for Veterinarians to test in their offices rather than sending out to a laboratory. Regardless of the cost, if you have a small dog, an older dog or are just concerned about your dog getting too much, a titer test is a good safety precaution, and the extra money you spend on the testing may be saved in the long run if your dog doesn't develop ill effects (tumors, cancer, kidney failure, neurological issues). For necessary vaccines, consider spacing them out, not having multiple injections at once and NEVER have your dog vaccinated when they are ill or recovering.

What we vaccinate against:

- BACTERIA – Bacteria are single-celled microorganisms that thrive in many different typesof environments. Some varieties live in extremes of cold or heat.
- VIRUS – Viruses are even smaller than bacteria and require living hosts - such as your pets or you --in order to multiply. When a virus enters your dog's body, it invades some of it's cells and takes over their normal function redirecting them to produce the virus.

The Vaccination:

- ANTIGEN – a substance that when introduced into a body triggers production of an antibody by stimulating the pet's immune system. Antigens prime the system to fight.

The Outcome:

- ANTIBODY – protein made by white blood cells that neutralize the effects of toxins; created in response to antigens and make pet immune to a specific disease.

Any medical procedure (including an injection) can have adverse side-effects, so watch your dog for several hours, even days, after any vaccination and get professional medical attention if any of the following arise:

- Fever
- Decrease in social behavior
- Diminished Appetite or Activity
- Sneezing
- Discomfort or swelling at injection site
- Swelling to face or legs
- Vomiting/Diarrhea
- Whole body itching
- Difficulty breathing
- Collapse

HOMEOPATHIC TIP: Thuja Occidentalis commonly known as Evergreen Conifer Tree, can aid with residual toxicity if given before and after vaccinations. See page 127 under Illness & Injuries to learn more about homeopathic therapies.

Core Vaccinations

Depending on where you live and what bacteria or viruses are in your region, additional vaccinations may be suggested by your Veterinarian, but as a rule, the following are considered the core inoculations dogs and cats should receive with a brief description of the diseases they protect against. Do note, that many illnesses have similar symptoms, so visit your Veterinarian for a professional diagnosis.
Dogs:

- Rabies
- DHLPP or DHPP (Distemper/Hepatitis/Leptospirosis/Parainfluenza/Parvovirus)
- Bordetella (important if your pet socializes with other dogs, gets boarded or even visits a veterinary office)

DOG DISEASES

If contracted, all of these preventable diseases require veterinary care, so protect your pets and keep an eye out for the earliest signs and symptoms. Unless noted, these diseases are species-specific and cannot spread from dog to cat to human. Those are covered under Zoonotic Diseases in this book. (See Page 55)

Canine Distemper virus can cause a variety of symptoms related to the central nervous system. Canine distemper is spread from dog to dog in secretions like saliva, urine and tears. It affects a variety of systems within the dog, such as the immune system (by suppressing the ability to make white blood cells and fight off infection), the central nervous system (resulting in seizures and erratic behavior), the gastrointestinal system (causing vomiting and diarrhea), and the respiratory system (resulting in coughing). Dogs that recover initially from the disease may have seizures or other central nervous system disorders later.

Symptoms:
- Lethargy
- Thick green eye discharge
- Seizures
- Vomiting and/or diarrhea

Preventive Measures: Vaccinate or confirm titers are high to insure immunity.

Hepatitis is a highly contagious viral disease that affects the liver, kidneys, lungs, spleen and eyes.

Early Symptoms:
- Lethargy
- Loss of appetite

Severe Symptoms:
- Fever
- Cough
- Swollen lymph nodes
- Jaundice
- Weight loss
- Dehydration, frequent thirst & urination
- Cloudy eyes
- Abdominal pain & swelling
- Pale tongue/gums
- Pale stool

Preventive Measures: Vaccinate or confirm titers are high to insure immunity.

Leptospirosis is a bacterial infection spread through urine and water sources. Typically rodents and wildlife are the carriers but dogs, cats, humans and other animals can become infected. Veterinary treatment is a must to prevent a public safety issue as well as for the health of the animal.

Symptoms:
- Fever
- Vomiting and/or diarrhea
- Muscle pain
- Jaundice of the inner ears, eyes and gums

Preventive Measures: Vaccinate or confirm titers are high to insure immunity. If Leptospirosis is not problematic in your area, the combo vaccine may be only a 4-in-1 DHPP as the Lepto vaccine is not considered necessary.

Parvovirus is a serious virus that attacks a dog's intestinal tract. It is so infectious that virtually anyone or any moving object can become a carrier simply by coming in contact with an infected dog's feces. Parvo can cause severe bloody diarrhea, vomiting, and electrolyte imbalances and can lead to severe dehydration, a buildup of toxins or poisons in the bloodstream, and eventually death. When puppies under 12 weeks old are infected, the virus can damage the heart muscle and cause lifelong cardiac problems. Though there are presently no drugs to kill the virus, there are treatments proven to control its symptoms.

Parvovirus can survive extreme heat and sub-zero temperatures for long periods of time, and can live on a surface (ie: sidewalk or kennel run) long after the feces has been removed. Use a solution of one part bleach to thirty parts water to clean areas frequented by other dogs, and use the solution on the soles of your shoes if you think you've walked through an infected area. Parvocide® is a good alternative to bleach.

Rottweilers, American Pit Bull Terriers, Doberman Pinchers, German Shepherds and English Springer Spaniels are more predisposed to Parvovirus, even when vaccinated, but no breed is immune. According to various studies, unvaccinated dogs are way more likely to contract Parvo than vaccinated dogs.

Symptoms:
- Vomiting and/or severe diarrhea
- Depression
- Loss of appetite

Preventive Measures: Most Veterinarians recommend multiple vaccinations for growing puppies to protect them from this virus. As dogs get older, their immunity is maintained with annual booster shots.

Canine Flu is a contagious viral infection of dogs caused by Influenza Virus A subtype H3N8. Canine influenza is an airborne disease, much like kennel cough. Physical contact between dogs does not seem to be required. Incubation time is approximately 2-5 days. It is a mutated strain that made the leap from horses to dogs but is not a mutation of Avian or Bird Flu which is a different subtype (H5N1). While both are in the same broad general family of viruses (Orthomyxoviridae) that cause the flu in people, pigs and birds, they are not the same strain.

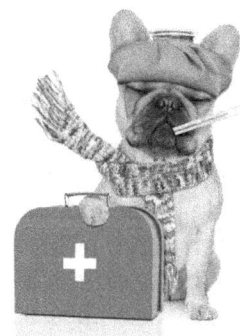

Typically, most infected dogs develop mild to moderate signs that resolve within 10-30 days without problems. They usually suffer from a persistent cough that may last for as long as three weeks and may experience a yellowish nasal discharge that can be treated effectively with antibiotics. As with other flu viruses, death can occur but is more commonly due to secondary complications such as pneumonia. Antibiotics are the most successful form of treatment.

Symptoms:
- Cough lasting weeks in spite of antibiotic treatment
- Nasal discharge
- Low-grade fever
- Loss of appetite
- Dehydration

What to do: Currently no vaccination exists. Contact your Veterinarian immediately. Be sure to tell your Veterinarian if your dog has been boarded, sent to the groomer or involved in any social activities (dog park, doggie day care, etc.) within the last month. Remember, coughing may be an indication of any variety of diseases. Your Veterinarian is best qualified to make the diagnosis. Keep your dog eating and well hydrated!

Kennel Cough (Bordetella bronchiseptica) is a very contagious upper respiratory infection that is passed from dog to dog at parks, day care centers, boarding facilities and shelters in particular.

Symptoms:
- Dry hacking cough (sounds like goose honking)
- Watery nasal discharge

Preventive Measures: Oral or Intranasal vaccination annually as the strain changes each year like our human flu vaccines do. Rarely do side effects occur from this vaccine. Veterinary treatment necessary if illness occurs.

Rabies is a rare disease in dogs in the United States, but whether you grew up on "Old Yeller" or "Cujo" you know it is very serious. Rabies affects the central nervous system and is classified as a virus. This virus is transmitted through the bite of a rabid mammal. The incubation period is about 30 to 60 days.

Once symptoms start, a usually friendly dog may become snappy or even ferocious. Foaming at the mouth is also a classic symptom. If you suspect your dog has rabies or has been bitten by an animal, take him to the vet immediately. If you are bitten by a rabid animal (bats, skunks & other animals can carry rabies), see your physician promptly for treatment. See page 55 under Zoonotic Diseases.

Preventive Measures: Vaccinate or confirm titers are high to assure immunity. Presently, rabies is a death sentence for our canine friends. Unfortunately more adverse side-effects occur from this vaccine than others, so be vigiant and consider all options to help boost your pets health. Do not give this vaccine at the same time your dog receives others (space them out by 2-4 weeks) and look for vaccines without mercury and other harmful preservatives. Learn more by visiting www.rabieschallengefund.org to get legislation passed so that too frequent vaccinations will no longer be required in order to legally license dogs in the U.S.

Heartworm Disease

What do San Francisco, Washington DC, and Las Vegas all have in common? They're all popular destinations for people – and heartworms. This disease is no longer confined to the southeast as dogs travel with their people and many east coast pooches have moved west in search of homes.

Heartworm disease is easy to prevent but hard and expensive to treat and can be fatal! Foot-long worms (heartworms) live in the heart, lungs and associated blood vessels of affected pets, causing severe lung disease, heart failure and damage to other organs in the body. Heartworm disease affects dogs, cats and ferrets, but heartworms also live in other mammals, in rare instances, humans! Dogs are a natural host for heartworms, which means that heartworms that live inside the dog, mature into adults, mate and produce offspring. Untreated, their numbers can increase, and dogs have been known to harbor several hundred worms in their bodies.

Heartworm disease causes lasting damage to the heart, lungs and arteries, and can affect the dog's health and quality of life long after the parasites are gone. For this reason, prevention is by far the best (and least expensive) option. Treatment however, should begin as early as the disease is detected and generally requires the dog to remain calm for the duration (approximately 6 months).

SIGNS & SYMPTOMS
Coughing
Weight Loss
Inactivity
Difficulty Breathing
Collapse

PREVENTIVE MEASURES:
The American Heartworm Society recommends:
> (1) get your pet tested every 12 months for heartworm and
> (2) give your pet heartworm preventive 12 months a year.

Zoonotic Diseases

Zoonotic diseases can be passed between species, meaning...YOU can get these from being around your pets. Zoonoses are infectious diseases that can be transmitted between animals and humans. Ebola, Zika & Hanta virus along with Swine & Bird flu may come to mind. HIV was a zoonotic disease transmitted to humans in the early 20th century but has now evolved into a separate human-only disease. In fact, 61% of the pathogens affecting humans are zoonotic! The increasing number and significance of zoonotic diseases emerging worldwide are due to multiple converging factors: climate change, increasing urbanization, human encroachment in wild areas, increased global travel and, for companion animals, increasing intimacy with humans (Yay! They are part of the family!) Zoonotic injuries include dog bites, cat scratches, tick and insect bites and stings, however...
Humans canNOT get Distemper from your canine pal any more than he can get Feline Rhinotracheitis from his kitty housemate. Knowing which diseases transfer between species and their signs and symptoms is vital if you share your life with animals, but also practice proper hygiene by thoroughly washing hands and wearing gloves when cleaning up after your best pal. The tiniest paper cut is bacteria's highway into your bloodstream!

Rabies – Vaccinate or confirm titers to prevent! Rabies is an acute and deadly viral infection of the central nervous system. Although rare in the United States for humans to actually contract rabies, 18,000 Americans each year get shots due to coming in contact with animals that may carry the disease. It is still quite prevalent in Third World Countries.

Giardia - Giardia & Coccidia are intestinal parasites that live in many animals. A dog can become infected by eathing the cyst form of the parasite when drinking from a pond, puddle or backyard water bucket that contains contaminated water. He can also pick it up eating the feces of other animals.

To prevent, provide pets with clean water and bowls and discourage them from eating feces. Also don't let them drink from communal bowls at dog parks, and bring along fresh water so that they don't lap out of lakes and streams. If in spite of your best attempts, massive quantities of vomit or diarrhea erupt, always wear rubber gloves when cleaning up and save those kisses for when your pooch is back in good health!

Preventive Measures: Because Giardia is not species-specific, people can get it from their pets or directly from contaminated water sources! Therefore, sanitation is of the utmost importance when caring for your dogs. Wear gloves when cleaning up feces, especially diarrhea or vomit from an infected animal, and wash your hands frequently when around your pets. The only sure way to prevent Giardia is to eliminate the source of the infection which is contaminated water as it can survive chlorination as well as frost. Any place water collects should be alleviated if possible such as places where there are puddles or poor drainage. Concrete surface should be cleaned, dried and sealed. Lysol®, ammonia or bleach (1% bleach, 99% water) can be effective decontamination agents, yet due to a protective outer shell, some Giardia survive chlorine treatments.

Signs & Symptoms:
- Diarrhea and/or vomitting
- Weight loss (Since Giardia prevent proper absorption of nutrients and interfere with digestion, your pet may lose weight in spite of eating a hearty meal.)

What to Do: Veterinary care is a must and humans should also get medical attention to get through the discomfort. Most common treatment is the drug Metronidazole (aka Flagyl) which cannot be given to pregnant pets or humans. Usually immunity to Giardia is not acquired after treatment, so contraction of the disease can re-occur. Prevention is always the best medicine, so at home, hiking or on vacation, be sure there is plenty of fresh water for Fido, Fluffy and you!

<u>Ringworm</u> is a fungus, not a worm! It gets its name from the appearance of a ring-shaped rash on the skin that is dry and scaly or wet and crusty with missing patches of hair or fur. Humans can acquire it from dogs and cats, puppies and kittens. Goats, cows, pigs and horses can transfer it to people as well. It can also be obtained from showers, pool surfaces and contaminated clothing. A Wood's Lamp (blue light) will make the fungus glow and determine diagnosis along with a skin biopsy or culture.

Preventive Measures: Prevent contact with infected animals so be on the look-out for signs and symptoms.

Signs & Symptoms:
- Red itchy & raised, scaly patches that may blister and ooze
- On humans, the patches are often redder on the outside with normal skin tone in the center making it appear like a clearly-defined ring.
- On pets, a circular patch of missing fur with a crusty center

What to do: Get pets to their Veterinarian for anti-fungal treatment and humans to their medical professionals! Ringworm is highly contagious!

To care for ringworm:
- Keep skin clean and dry.
- Apply antifungal or drying powders, lotions, or creams that contain miconazole, clotrimazole, or whatever is prescribed by your medical professional.
- Don't wear clothing that rubs against and irritates the area.
- Wash sheets and night clothes, dog bedding every day while infected exists in your household.

Tick-Borne Diseases

Lyme Disease (measles-like eruptions accompanied by muscle aches, nausea and swollen lymph nodes) and Rocky Mountain Spotted Fever ('target'-shaped rash bringing with it headache and nausea) are both tick-borne diseases. Keep pets free of parasites and check yourself after hikes.

NEWLY EMERGING TICK DISEASES…
American canine hepatozoonosis (ACH) is highly debilitating and often fatal! The disease is spread not from the bite of ticks but rather by dogs ingesting infected nymphal or adult Gulf Coast ticks.

Signs & Symptoms:
- Abnormally large increase in the number of white blood cells during acute infection or inflammation (Leukocytosis)
- Abnormal growth of soft the tissue (periosteum) which lines the outside of the long bones in dogs,
- Fever
- Depression
- Muscle pain, atrophy & weakness
- Weight loss
- Prognosis only 1-2 years

Anaplasmosis is a bacterial disease that presents in two forms in dogs and is on the rise:
- Anaplasma phagocytophilium infects white blood cells (this is the form that is also found in people) – transmitted by the deer tick and western black-legged tick and since these two ticks are also vectors for other diseases, it is not uncommon for dogs to be co-infected with Erhlichia, Rocky Mountain spotted fever and/or Lyme disease.
- Anaplasma platys, infects a dog's platelets – transmitted by the brown dog and lone star tick

The areas with greatest incidence are the northeastern states, Gulf states, California, upper Midwest, southwestern states, and mid-Atlantic regions.

Signs & Symptoms:
 usually begin within one to two weeks of the initial bite, but vary depending on which organism has infected the dog.

Reported signs in **A. phago** include:
- Lameness and joint pain
- Lethargy
- Loss of appetite
- Fever
- Less commonly: coughing, seizures, vomiting and diarrhea

A. platys infects the platelets, which are responsible for blood clotting, so signs are related to the body's inability to properly stop bleeding and include:

- Bruising
- Red splotches on the gums and belly
- Nosebleeds

Blood and platelet testing is imperative to determine.

Babesiosis is caused by a bite from the black-legged tick. Incubation averages two weeks but symptoms are often mild and go undiagnosed for years resulting immune-mediated hemolytic anemia, where the red blood cells (RBCs) are broken down and hemoglobin is released into the body. This can lead to jaundice and to anemia.

Signs & Symptoms:
- Lack of energy
- Lack of appetite leading to weight loss
- Pale mucous membranes
- Fever
- Icterus/Jaundice
- Enlarged Lymph Nodes and Spleen
- May also affect multiple organ systems
- Shock & collapse

Pregnant moms can pass on to pups or kittens. Greyhounds, pit bull terriers, and American Staffordshire terriers seem to be most susceptible to infection.

Being vigilant about tick avoidance and removal is the best method for preventing ALL tick-borne diseases!

The Importance of Spaying & Neutering

For every human being born, approximately 15 puppies are born. How can we possibly provide them all safe and loving forever homes? Dogs generally only have 2 cycles annually, but due to litter size, one non-spayed canine and her offspring can produce 67,000 dogs in only seven years!

Many animals die giving birth when bred before 6 months of age as they are still babies themselves. In the case of large-headed breeds (pugs and bulldogs for instance), many pups are too large to be delivered naturally, and if they are not delivered by Caesarean, with the help of a Veterinarian, both the mom and pups can die.

Pet overpopulation is the number one killer of pets! Every 11 seconds a dog or cat is euthanized in the United States. With 80,000 pets born each day versus only 10,000-15,000 people, there will never be enough humans to care for them. Limiting their population growth is the best way to prevent animal homelessness, curb certain diseases, and keep our pets safe.

Spaying and neutering can decrease AGGRESSIVENESS in many pets as hormones no longer rage since the source of their production has been removed. However, your pet still remains protective of his home and family as if he was prior to surgery.

Spay/neuter can decrease SPRAYING (urine marking) particularly by male cats who no longer feel the need to mark their territory. It can also decrease an animal's desire to roam in search of a mate and therefore, your pet stays safely at home. Studies show that 80% of all pets hit by cars are unneutered males!

Spaying females can lower their risks of mammary and uterine cancer as well as pyometra (an infection of the uterus that can erupt into an emergency situation).

Neutering males can lower prostate issues, so just check with your Veterinarian to find out what age is best to have your pet altered. Most animals go home the same day as surgery and suffer no ill effects (as long as you prevent them from picking at their stitches).

- In brief, SPAYING (ovariohysterectomy) includes the removal of the ovaries, fallopian tubes and uterus. General anesthesia is necessary.

- NEUTERING removes the testicles but will allow your dog to retain his own unique personality. General anesthesia is required, but neuter patients recover more quickly than their female counterparts as neutering is not considered major surgery since it is not performed deep in the abdominal cavity. Non-surgical neutering is in development, so stay tuned to breakthroughs.

Confirm local laws as spay/neuter may decrease the COST OF LICENSING in your area or may actually be mandatory at a certain age for all pets. Low cost clinics and vouchers from humane organizations are available to help those having difficulty paying for spay/neuter surgery. In the long run, the medical cost is much cheaper than caring for a litter of puppies or kittens.

Common Myths Dispelled
Spaying/Neutering DOES NOT make your dog fat or lazy – lack of exercise and overfeeding does.

Dogs DO NOT need to have one litter to settle down. Having a litter will not improve your dog's health or change their personality. Actually, pregnancy and nursing can sometimes cause dogs to become tired & irritable.

DON'T leave your dog unaltered so that your child can see the "miracle of birth." Most pets hide when giving birth and even if you find good homes for your litter, you may deny homes to animals that have already been born. There are plenty of videos available to learn these life lessons.

CARING FOR A NEONATE: Your Newborn Puppy

Red Flags
Seek IMMEDIATE medical attention if your puppy is:
- Coughing
- Sneezing
- Gagging
- Wheezing

Has:

- Diarrhea
- Vomiting
- Loss or increased appetite
- Change in behavior

Is:

- Twitching abnormally
- Straining to urinate or defecate
- Tiring easily
- Breathing heavily
- Bleeding from any part of the body

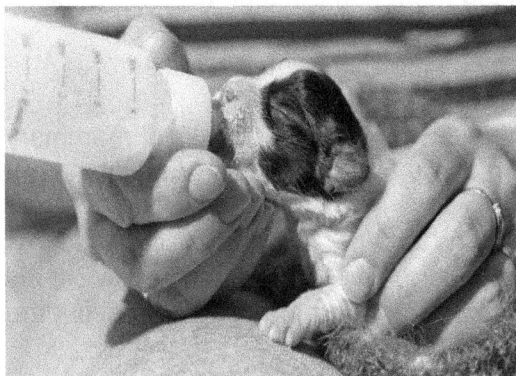

Milestones:
Week #1	Weight should double
Week #2	Eyes open! If they seem weepy or pus-filled, gently wipe with a warm, wet, soft cloth but do not pry open. Let eyes open naturally. Fur babies can hear!
Week #3	Crawling on all fours!
Week #4	Puppies begin playing with each other and start to develop teeth. Ouch! The transition begins to wet food.
Week #6	Dry food is on the menu and eye color may begin changing from blue (although true color doesn't settle in until about the 3rd month).

Warmth
Keeping your newborn puppy warm is of supreme importance. Neonates haven't yet developed the ability to keep themselves temperate so they are very dependent on you for their climate control. Being too hot or too cold can be a true medical emergency!

Cleanliness
No animal can stay healthy if he is not kept clean. Puppies will soil themselves.
If you have a litter, the animals will groom each other, and if feces, old food or mucous is stuck in their fur, the other animal will ingest it and become ill.

Bathe puppies carefully in warm water using puppy shampoo taking care not to get water or shampoo in their eyes, ears, nose or mouth. Always use species specific products (do not use soaps, flea preventatives, or anything for dogs that is made for cats). After the bath, wrap the pet in a towel and dry thoroughly. This also creates a loving bond between you and your baby canine.

Feeding

Never feed a newborn when he or she is cold as they are prone to aspiration pneumonia, gut motility problems and won't be able to properly digest their food. Warm fluids should be administered until the animal is warm enough to be fed.

An eye dropper or bottle with nipple will be needed for a puppy who does not have a mom to nurse him. Use a sewing needle or a 16-18 gauge hypodermic needle to first pierce the tip of the nipple. Too large of an opening in the nipple could cause the pup to aspirate the fluid into the lungs. Too small of an opening will prevent him from getting the nutrition he needs.

Before you begin feeding, thoroughly clean the bottle and nipple in hot water and wash your hands with antibacterial soap. Gently open the puppy's mouth with the tip of your finger and gently slip the nipple in. You will feel a vacuum effect when he gets the nipple into suckle mode and will probably then hold on enthusiastically. Keep the bottle at a 45 degree angle with light tension on the bottle to prevent air from getting into the young one's stomach.

If the puppy refuses the bottle, try rubbing his forehead or back to simulate how his mom would clean him and encourage him to nurse.

Let him suck at his own pace but do not overfeed – animals generally let you know when they've had enough. Each feeding can take 20-30 minutes via the bottle. If the animal is choking, immediately and carefully hold him upside down. Below is a good rule of thumb to follow for small breed puppies. Increase for larger breeds:

Newborn to 1 week old	1 – 2 Tablespoons
1 – 2 weeks	3 Tablespoons
2 – 3 weeks	4 – 5 Tablespoons
3 – 4 weeks	6 Tablespoons

Make only enough formula that will be used within 48 hours. For canned formula, freeze any leftovers in an ice cube tray and thaw only what you need for each additional feeding. Pet Ag makes Esbilac® for puppies. Cow's milk is not a good substitute for young dogs.

Puppies sometimes need to be encouraged to defecate. Momma dogs help their kids along by licking their babies' urogenital openings to stimulate urination and defecation. If you are playing the role of mom, use a cotton ball dampened with warm water to wipe the areas. Remember to wash your hands before and after handling neonates. Always use clean towels and don't believe the old wives tale about newspaper being sterile, unless it is non-inked! The ink from newspaper can be toxic and easily absorbed through the animal's skin.

Like humans, canines are about 70% water and need to stay well-hydrated. Daily test their hydration by gently pulling up on the skin at the nape of their neck and releasing. This is called the skin tugor test, and a well-hydrated animal's skin will snap back quickly – within one second or less. If the skin stays in a peak or takes 2-3 seconds to return to position, give fluids through a needle-less syringe or eye dropper and seek medical attention immediately.

At Four Weeks

At four weeks, pups should now be fed every 4-6 hours transitioning to wet/canned/soft food. They should also start drinking water on their own at this time. Often puppies start biting at their bottle nipple when they are ready for this change. To encourage your puppy to eat wet food, Esbilac® with the soft food into a porridge-like consistency and serve off a spoon or your finger until they are ready to plunge into their food bowl. At this stage of the game they still lack coordination and often fall head first into their food bowls so be prepared to clean your little one after each meal and don't be surprised if he or she treats you to spells of diarrhea during this weaning period.

At Six Weeks

Another food transition and yes...more diarrhea comes at 6 weeks of age when you should wean your puppy from the soft food to dry food. For the first week, mix canned and dry together and gradually reduce the amount of wet. Make sure you are using puppy kibble so that the bits are small enough to be chewed by teeny weenie teeth. By 8 weeks the kibble size may be increased, especially for large breed puppies, as long as they are able to chew the bits comfortably – you do not want a choking incident.

Socializing

Emotional and physical closeness is important to puppies. Let them snuggle, pet them as much as you can, and try out various toys to find out which ones stimulate their brain power and develop their motor skills. As they reach 6-8 weeks old, they should be out of their crates more safely exploring the world WITH YOU. Let them walk about a bedroom or other smaller room where you can keep a watchful eye. Make sure cords and strings are out of paws reach but let them use their muscles and gain control of their motor skills while smelling the scents of home. Make sure there are no chemicals or cleaning products on the floor, and watch that they don't slip between furniture or escape from the house completely.

"We adopted a 6-week old Retriever mix at a time in our life when we just weren't interacting with a lot of people," Lucy Johnson of Leesburg, Florida shares. "On the rare occasion when someone would stop by, we'd have to shut Blossom in a back bedroom because she would go ballistic growling at the stranger." Socialize early to avoid problems.

There is nothing as cute as a bundle of fur licking your face with that distinct puppy breath and a soft round tummy. It can turn any grown-up into a cooing human child. Rediscovering the world through an inquisitive puppy's eyes is a delight, but it's also important to note how first experiences must be good and positive for your young one. A hand or voice raised in anger or a lack of experiences with others can allow a doggone adorable pooch to grow into a dog of questionable temperament. From the moment your puppy enters your life, you must socialize her to become a friendly and confident dog.

According to the American Veterinary Society of Animal Behavior (AVSAB), "The primary and most important time for puppy socialization is the first three months of life. During this time, puppies should be exposed to as many new people, animals, stimuli and environments as can be achieved safely" to make them aware and unafraid of the world.
"A puppy at two months of age is equivalent to a 14-month old infant...

while a dog at 6 months is like a 5-year old child!" explains Caroline Haldeman, owner of Sirius K9 Training Academy in Yorba Linda, California. "Often new dog owners are told by their Veterinarians that they must keep their dog confined until he is finished with his vaccinations. What they should be told instead is how dogs catch disease and how you can socialize them safely."

Well-run puppy classes strive to desensitize puppies that would otherwise be kept at home. Inspired by how well the guide dogs she raised became socialized, San Fernando Valley California dog trainer Laurie King turned her home tennis court into a special place for puppies and their people to meet each other. In class the pups are held while experiencing a variety of sights, sounds and textures, but they also are required to sit quietly while pet owners share behavior issues as well as develop realistic expectations of their dog.

Positive reinforcement-based training is also a key component in turning out well-adjusted pets. "The benefits are positively huge," says Ian Dunbar, Director of the Center for Applied Animal Behavior in Berkeley, California. "Puppies learn bite inhibition through puppy play and proper interaction with people during off-leash play and while being handled by strangers."

"When pups are small, finger nibbling may be cute, but when your large puppy -- weighing in at 50+ pounds -- body slams you, it's not so funny," says Susan Barnes of Scottsdale, Arizona of her Rotties. "Stopping undesirable behavior in its tracks keeps me safe and my dogs well-homed."

A dog that is not properly socialized can develop fear issues as well as an inability to cope with changes in his environment. This can result in problems for owners, Veterinarians and groomers alike when they try to examine, handle or even come near the dog. Severely under-socialized animals can remain fearfully aggressive for life making them unsuitable as pets, and shelters are filled with good dogs that humans didn't take the time to train and properly socialize.

The main risk for attending a group class at an early age would be disease, but the American College of Veterinary Behaviorists (ACVB) states, "We are aware of only one Parvo problem in a puppy preschool class in Minnesota in the early 90s and none since high titer Parvo vaccines gained mainstream use in 1995. There have also been no puppy class participants infected with Parvovirus in any puppy classes offered at Ohio State or Purdue University."

Most dogs get sick from coming in contact with other dogs' urine or feces. Keeping your less than four-month-old pup away from public grass and water greatly decreases her chance of contracting disease. Class locations should bleach surfaces and quickly clean up accidents. "The true danger period is around 12 weeks of age when most maternal immunity is gone and the pup's own immunity has not kicked in yet," says Deb Eldredge, DVM in Vernon, New York. At this time due diligence is vital, so expose your puppy to only healthy dogs.

"I recommend a series of vaccinations (Distemper, Parvovirus, Parinfluenza, and Hepatitis) starting at 7 weeks and continuing approximately every 3 weeks until a dog is 16 weeks old. Bordetella is usually given near the end of the series while the Rabies vaccination is given at 4 months," explains Dr. Liz Koskenmaki of Media City Animal Hospital in Burbank, California. She also suggests deworming puppies and obtaining a clean fecal test prior to interaction with others.

"In fact, the risk of a dog dying because of infection is far less than the much higher risk of a dog being euthanized due to a behavior problem," states DVM Robert K. Anderson, University of Minnesota. A few precautions paired with sensible canine interaction can go a long way towards getting your puppy off on the right paw to a long, happy life with you!

People and the Human Touch

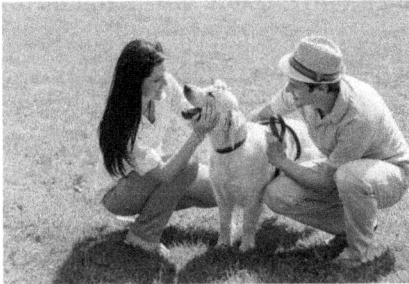

People are number one on the list as far as "what" you should desensitize your puppy to according to Vernon, New York Veterinarian Deb Eldredge, "and people of different sizes, ages, sexes, people with hats, people with facial hair." She insists that every new thing should be positive. "Give a scary tall man with a beard a treat as he approaches your puppy," she suggests.

Uniforms sometimes cause a stir, so have the letter carrier, package delivery service and meter reader all make friends with your pet. Their safety is important as well as your pup's, so teach him to not act aggressively towards these individuals when they enter your property.

Dog Mom Norma Chavez says, "I took a Pet First-Aid Class and learned the importance of doing a weekly head-to-tail check-up on my German Shepherd. Bella became so used to me touching her that it's now easy if she gets hurt, needs a bath or has to be touched for any reason. She'll let me feel around and even put an ice pack on her. I never had a dog before that was used to this."

By enrolling in a puppy class, your dog gets off on the right paw of being used to other healthy well-mannered animals. Continue that habit throughout his lifetime, but chose your pup's role models wisely

Sights, Sounds and Smells

At home, pull out the vacuum cleaner, ring the doorbell, clap your hands and play the stereo. Pop some corn or percolate coffee with your furry angel by your side. Strap him into a doggie seat belt and take him for short car rides letting him hear motorcycles and screeching tires. Place him in a wagon (if you don't yet want paws touching public space) and stroll him through neighborhoods and outdoor malls. Don't forget his favorite toy and treats to turn a scary bicyclist or skate boarder into a new friend. Walk by a senior center or hospital so she can experience a walker or wheel chair. Remember his perspective (6" – 20" inches off the ground) is different from yours and fear must be overcome to prevent skittishness as fearful pets may become aggressive. Bring him to the Veterinarian just to sit and receive a treat and don't forget to let him experience rain, lakes and even snow under your watchful supervision but don't take him to fireworks displays. Life happens. Make it fun for your dog but keep it safe!

The Carrier/Crate

The purpose of a dog carrier/crate is really three-fold…it is a den to keep the animal safe, helps with potty training and allows them to develop a tolerance for the carrier for later life, like going to the Veterinarian!

Since young dogs and cats aren't yet equipped to control their body temperature, placing a heating pad on a low setting in the carrier conserves the warmth keeping the animal comfortable. The heating pad should be well wrapped in a towel with another towel on top of it – the puppy should NEVER make contact with the pad directly and should be used only until the animal is about 4 weeks old. Constantly recheck your heating pad for safety sake!

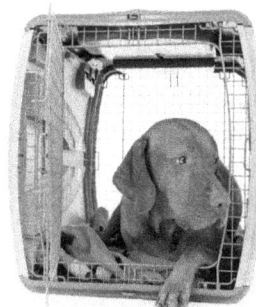

Carriers/crates should be kept in draft-free locations and the bedding will need to be changed several times daily. By four weeks when they are transitioning to wet food, start putting the puppy outside on leash with you immediately after each meal to train them where to go.

PET SAFETY

You can't keep your pet in a plastic bubble – life happens, and statistics show that 9 out of 10 pets are going to experience an emergency at some point during their lifetime, so don't be caught not knowing what to do. Although tips are provided in this section, more detailed first-aid techniques are available in the back of this book to walk you through what to do when the worst happens.

Beforehand, make your pet's environment as safe as possible and always keep your eyes wide open. When you have a dog, you have a furry toddler for life, and…one who possesses a PAWmazing sense of smell! This means that even when you may feel items are put away, they are never truly out of "paws reach" if they smell good enough to get. Our dogs can smell a whole lot better than we can – statistics show their sense of smell is from 1,000 to 1,000,000 times better than ours! Think of it this way…You and your dog stroll out the front door (on-leash of course) towards the mailbox. You notice a neighbor is cooking stew for dinner. Then as you reach the street, you smell exhaust from a passing car.

Finally, as you open the mailbox, you bend down to smell the sweet scent of the rose planted next to it. That's about it for our human sniffers. Fido, however, has been on over-drive since coming out the door! As he walks beside you down the front path, he is nose to the ground smelling every critter that has crossed since the last rain. If he even bothers to lift his head, he doesn't smell the neighbor's stew – he smells beef, carrots, onions, potatoes, rosemary, garlic and every individual ingredient in the recipe. Upon reaching the mailbox, exhaust is of no importance to your pooch. He is zeroing in on the urine left behind by the local canines. He can tell if it's a male and how tall he is by the height of the pee stream as well as if the female is in heat. If he bothers with the rose bush, each petal and leaf smell a bit different depending on whether they are new or in a state of decay, whether a bee or butterfly has recently landed upon one. At long last when you pull out the mail, your dog can smell everyone who has touched the envelope on its journey to you and if he could speak our language, he could tell you what the person who licked the envelope had for dinner! This means that an item of no concern to us has a virtual rainbow of scents to our pet, and if tempting enough, your dog or cat might seek it out.

Down on all fours
Look at life from your dog's perspective. What may be perfectly tidy at 5'4", 6'2" or wherever you stand…is a whole different world at 6" - 24" off the floor. Anything on the floor is fair game, so besides teaching dogs "no" and "leave it," it is up to you to limit the dangers they can encounter.

K9 Chaos
The following are some of the many common items to keep out of paws reach in basic home scenarios:

Living Room
- Electric cords
- TV – remote controls can look like toys
- Stereos – can be deafeningly loud to animals' sensitive hearing
- Falling knick knacks, pictures, lamps
- Sharp coffee table edges
- Cords from blinds and draperies – choking and entanglement issues
- Rug chewing – result in intestinal blockages
- Rocking chairs – can catch tails and paws
- Fireplace including smokeless logs from which the sawdust can cause a bowel obstruction and lighter fluid poisoning
- Heating units/vents

Kitchen

According to the Pet Poison Helpline® (800) 213-6680, the Top 10 Kitchen Toxins are:

1) Chocolate
2) Grapes, raisins, currants
3) Xylitol found in sugar-free gum & candy
4) Fatty table scraps
5) Onions & garlic
6) Compost
7) Human Medications
   - NSAIDs (Advil, Aleve & Motrin for example)
   - Acetaminophen (Tylenol)
   - Antidepressants (Effexor, Cymbalta, Prozac, Lexapro)
   - ADD/ADHD Medications (Adderall, Ritalin, Concerta)
   - Benzodiazepines & Sleep Aids (Xanax, Klonopin, Ambien, Lunesta)
   - Birth Control (Estrogen, Estradiol, Progesterone)
   - ACE Inhibitors (Zestril, Altace)
   - Beta Blockers (Tenormin, Toprol, Coreg)
   - Thyroid Hormones (Armour desiccated thyroid, Synthroid)
   - Cholesterol Lowering Agents (Lipitor, Zocor, Crestor)
8) Macadamia Nuts
9) Cleaning Supplies
10) Unbaked bread dough & alcohol, both of which can lead to alcohol poisoning

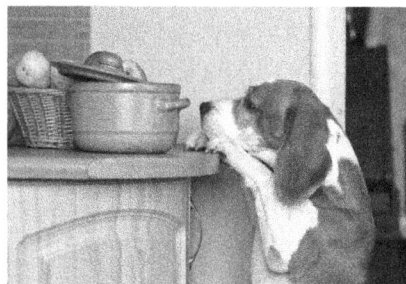

But also watch out for…

- Stove/Oven – not only can they be hot, but can Rover push buttons or turn knobs?
- Electric cords & outlets – can be enticing if splashed by food items
- Cleaners
- Other pantry items – many are fatal to pets (see page 235 for list of common poisonous foods) Oxygen absorbers placed in meat packing containers
- Knives and sharp tools
- Cabinet doors/refrigerator/dishwasher – make sure pets don't get closed in tight quarters and food gets dropped – pets can be stepped on

Bathroom

- Medications -- #1 cause of poisoning in our pets! Prescription & over the counter.
- Medical Marijuana (but of course this could be "stashed" elsewhere in the home)
- Cleaners
- Falling in or drinking out of toilet containing chemicals
- Electric outlets and appliances
- Candles
- Standing water in tubs or showers which could be a drowning hazard
- Dental Floss

Bedroom

- Drapery and blind cords
- Anything that can fall – knick knacks, pictures, mirrors, television sets, items from shelves
- Bed collapse – if pet sleeps underneath
- Rug or blanket chewing
- Any medications in nightstand
- Batteries (such as from hearing aids or other appliances)
- Getting closed in cabinets/closets
- Children's toys which could be anywhere in the house
- Shoe laces, hair ribbons and other such pieces of clothing

Garage & Outdoor Areas

- Paints, paint removers, cleaners of all types
- Insecticides & fertilizers
- Car engines – always tap on in cold months as an animal could be keeping warm near the engine and check before you back out!
- Barbeques – charcoal, lighter fluid, matches and the flame itself
- Fences – are they tall enough, can your pet dig under, is there anything close enough for him to jump on and then over the fence, are boards tight fitting with no sharp edges or nails protruding? Is fence-fighting a concern with a neighbor dog? A solid barrier may be needed.
- Gates – secure with not too large of a gap under or at closure for pet to squeeze through? Dog House or Kennel – sharp edges, well-ventilated, no parasites
- Pools/Spas/Fountains – drowning is always a concern; fenced off or ALWAYS supervise pets! What about chlorine and other chemicals? If pet gets into or drinks water containing chemicals, either could be very bad news.
- Sprinkler systems and outdoor electrical wiring
- Hot concrete and other surfaces
- Trash – secured lids
- Wildlife – pet friendly deterrents may be needed to keep them away; motion sensor lighting & sprinklers; picking up trash & dropped fruit to avoid raccoons or opossums; citronella and pet-safe preventives from mosquitoes, fleas and ticks

While this is not a complete list, it is a great starting point for you. Please take time to review your entire home for potential issues and problems.

Besides locations, each season has its own inherent dangers to our dogs. Fun-in-the-sun, splash-in-the-pool, throw-one-on-the-barbie time can be dangerous for your pets unless you keep a watchful eye. Cookouts can result in burned paws while summer-time foods like burgers, franks and fried chicken can cause canine pancreatitis (an inflammation of the organ that is the body's source of insulin and enzymes necessary for digestion).

Spring & Summer

Warmer weather, blooming plants and buzzing insects can spell trouble for your dogs but also note that depending where you live, winter hazards may still apply.

Observe your dogs in the yard, on a hike or at the lake. Dangers exist everywhere, but good pet parenting can prevent disasters and fix up minor injuries.

Insects

If your playful pooch gets stung by a bee, scrape away the stinger if you actually see it in his fur coat (or on his nose, lip or paw). Pulling the stinger with fingers or tweezers could rupture the poison sac allowing the toxin to enter your pet's body. Next administer 1 mg Benadryl® (Diphenhydramine) per pound of your pet's body weight, and apply a cold pack for short periods at a time (a bag of frozen peas works well) to any swelling. Remove ice pack frequently so as not to cause frostbite to the tissue or discomfort to your pet in general. If the swelling is severe or if any breathing difficulties develop, get to your Veterinarian at once! (Reference page 146 for more information)

Rising Temperatures

Be sure dogs have plenty of shade and water as it warms up but realize colder days sometimes revisit. Know weather patterns and stay alert to your regional changes.

Dogs don't sweat! Panting works like an evaporative cooling system bringing in cool air only if there is any. An air-conditioned house is safest for your pet, but the next best thing is a well ventilated / insulated doghouse or a shaded porch with a fan or misting system. Provide fresh water all day long making sure that outside bowls remain in the shade even when the sun moves in the late afternoon. You don't want the heat beating down on the water when your best friend is at his thirstiest.

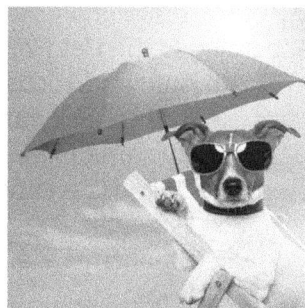

Bowls that attach to a hose and an outdoor spigot to continuously refill are preferable. Some dogs cool their paws in the bowl splashing the water out. By just supplying a larger bowl or tub, it becomes a bird bath and then water is not potable. Make sure water is in clean supply all day, everyday.

Tap water and many bottled waters are full of contaminants that a simple filter can remove. Heavy metals, chlorine and pharmaceuticals are just some of the toxins found in water. They can affect your dog's skin, coat and overall health! Always, always use either a stainless steel, glass or ceramic bowl for water. Plastic bowls can leach toxins into the water so avoid them altogether. Place outside food bowls in a pan containing a few inches of water to keep ants at bay. Notice the sun's patterns in regards to shade as well. Trees may not have grown their full complement of leaves by the time the sun is burning down. Also, as that fireball in the sky moves, it could be casting shade only on the other side of your fence, out of your dog's comfort zone. Fresh water and plenty of shade is a must for your dog at all times!

Hot concrete and asphalt can burn precious paws! Walk your dogs during the cool parts of the day and stick to the grass, even sand can burn paws. If it's too hot for your bare feet, it's too hot for paws. Dog shoes are great on hot surfaces for short periods of time, but since heat is expelled from the pads of the feet, your dog is likely to overheat if his paws are covered for long.

When out for a car ride, if your pet cannot go with you on every stop, leave him at home in a comfortable environment. Even with windows open, a parked car can quickly reach more than 150°F resulting in heat stroke, permanent brain damage or death to your pet. Never EVER leave your dog unattended in the car for even a few minutes. Additionally, they could be dog-napped or badly injured by shattered glass if someone tries to break into your car.

Plants
It is important to learn which plants in your yard are poisonous. Besides the toxins that flowers, bulbs, leaves and stems contain, thorns can cause pain and infections. Many fruits and vegetables can also be problematic. Remember, canine and human bodies are not the same, and just because we eat it does not make it safe for our dogs. Keep grapes and raisins, onions and chives, seeds and fruit pits away from Fido – the stone pit or seed in fruits such as peaches and plums contain an arsenic or cyanide-like substance that can prove fatal.

According to the Pet Poison Helpline®, the 10 most dangerous plants to our pets are:
- Autumn Crocus – all parts
- Azalea – all parts
- Cyclamen – all parts
- Daffodils – especially bulbs
- Diffenbachia – leaves and stems
- Kalanchoe – all parts including vase water are toxic
- Lilies – true lilies…Tiger, Asiatic, Easter and Japanese Snow can be fatal to cats! Others may cause milder symptoms.
- Oleander – all parts, even the water in a vase, are toxic
- Sago Palm – all parts but seeds most deadly
- Tulips/Hyacinths – especially bulbs

Find a more comprehensive list on page 235.

Also take caution with what you put on your plants…fertilizers, insecticides and even yard trimmings can be fatal if ingested by your pet. Have phone numbers accessible for your Veterinarian and Poison Control (ASPCA Animal Poison Control # - 888-426-4435), and know where your nearest animal emergency center is located. In an emergency, you don't want to be looking up directions!

Try this pet friendly weed killer you can make yourself:
>   1 Gallon White Vinegar
>   2 Cups Epsom Salts
>   ¼ Cup Dawn® Dish Soap (the original blue works best)
>   Mix and spray in the morning after the dew has evaporated.
>   By dinner time…weeds are gone!

Also realize organic fertilizers can be deadly if consumed. Blood meal is flash frozen blood that has been dried and ground but is still found tasty to pets. Often it is infused with iron resulting in a toxic overdose if Fido consumes while bone meal is made from animal bones that have been ground to powder. That meaty taste is inviting but when ingested, can form a large concrete-like ball in your dog's stomach which requires surgical removal.

Water Fun
Don't assume your dog can swim! Many animals drown each year, so install a fence or pool alarm and teach your furry friends how to get out of the pool by guiding them to the steps or a ramp. Review this lesson often, and if you take your dog to the lake or on a boat, put him in a life vest and watch paws for fish hooks, sharp rocks and other dangers. Safely store all chemicals associated with your pool and outdoor activities such as chlorine, pH, diatomaceous earth for filters and do not let the pool become your dog's drinking bowl since you add these chemicals to the water. Remember that pool toys can make a pet curious causing him to jump in unattended or even get entangled or choke on chewed pieces. It pays to know dog first-aid every season of the year, because harm can and could happen to your pet. Be prepared for the sake of Fido!

Along with the most obvious concern of drowning, be in-the-know about a condition called hyponatremia in which a swimming, diving or ball retrieving dog can consume too much water, unbalancing potassium levels and leading to death. See page 221.

By being an always alert dog parent, you can keep the fun flowing while keeping your furry kids out of harm's way, so open your eyes to impending hazards that could put on the brakes to summer-time fun.

Parasites, Insects & Snakes
Control fleas and ticks and keep your pets well groomed, but don't shave long-haired pets down to the skin as their fur insulates from the heat and prevents sunburn. Learn dog first-aid for bee stings and insect bites. Hot weather brings out rattlesnakes. Your best safety device is keeping control of your dog by having him on a leash. Limit the rodent population in your yard by removing ivy and piles of wood since where there are mice, there are snakes to eat them! Should your dog get bitten by a rattlesnake, keep him calm and immediately transport him to an animal care center that carries antivenin. See pages 145 - 155 before you need to know what you must do for snake bites and bee stings.

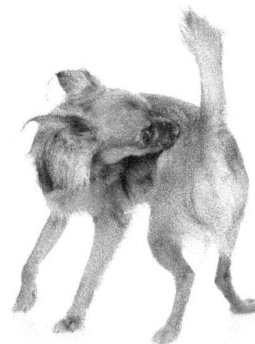

Paws Off

Keep insect repellents and sunscreens out of reach. If ingested by your dog, these products can result in neurological problems, vomiting and diarrhea. This includes citronella candles and other such items.

Make sure your pets keep paws and claws off matches and lighter fluid. Some matches contain chlorates which if ingested by Fido can damage his red blood cells, cause difficulty breathing or even kidney problems. Lighter fluid can irritate the skin, cause gastrointestinal, central nervous system, and pulmonary distress.

Also, since the hot days have arrived, make sure your pet doesn't walk on any surfaces that could burn his paws. If it's too hot for your bare feet, it's too hot for Fido's four paws! Be aware of the dangers of heat stroke and make sure your pets have plenty of cool, fresh water and shade to retreat to. Getting over heated can result in permanent brain damage and death to your pet, so never, never, never leave him alone in a parked car -- even for a short time. It only takes a few minutes (with the windows rolled down which can present a danger in itself) for the car to heat to deadly temperatures. See Heatstroke on page 189.

When the day is done, you'll be happy to have taken extra care so that your dogs will be around to spend many long and happy years by your side.

Fall, Winter & Colder Days to Come
A sudden change of schedule can lead to stress in your dog and can cause behavioral problems. Extra attention and a new friend may be the solution.

After a summer of playing ball, swimming, catching fireflies and getting lots of attention from his favorite boy or girl, your dog may not be himself when the kids dash off on the first day of the new school year. The sudden disruption to his schedule and quality time may cause your pet to eat too much, not want to eat at all or start eating strange objects such as plants, dirt, toys or clothing. This can result in vomiting, diarrhea and skin problems or more. Now is the time to give your four-legged family member some extra attention and to sharpen up on your pet first-aid and CPR skills because no matter how hard you try...life happens.

As leaves begin to fall, gardening tools and other sharp objects may get hidden. Look around to be sure that nothing can cut precious paws.

Don't leave dogs outdoors when the temperature drops. Most dogs are safer indoors, except when taken out for exercise. Regardless of the season, shorthaired, very young, or old dogs should never be left outside without supervision. Short-coated dogs may feel more comfortable wearing a sweater during walks. If your dog is an outdoor dog, he must be protected by a dry, draft-free doghouse that is large enough to allow the dog to sit and lie down comfortably, but small enough to hold in his/her body heat. The floor should be raised a few inches off the ground and covered with cedar shavings or straw. The house should be faced away from the wind, and the doorway should be covered with waterproof burlap or heavy plastic. Dogs who spend a lot of time outdoors need more food in the winter since trying to keep warm depletes energy. Frequently check your dog's water dish to make certain the water is fresh and unfrozen. Use bacteria resistant food and water bowls. Keep in mind; when the temperature is low, your pet's tongue can stick and freeze to metal.

Warm engines in parked cars attract cats and small wildlife who may crawl up under the hood to get warm. To avoid injuring any hidden animals, bang on your car's hood to scare them away before starting your engine.

Salt and other chemicals used to melt snow and ice can irritate the pads of your dog's feet. Wipe paws gently with a damp towel before your dog licks them and irritates his mouth. Antifreeze is a deadly poison, but it has a sweet taste that attracts animals. Take care to quickly wipe up spills and store antifreeze (and all household chemicals) out of reach. Better yet, use antifreeze-coolant made with propylene glycol; if swallowed in small amounts, it should not hurt dogs.

HOLIDAYS

New Year's Resolutions for Your Dog

I RESOLVE TO:
Do a weekly head-to-tail check-up of my dog and really get acquainted with his habits so that I can discover a small problem before it becomes a nightmare.

Schedule a visit with our Veterinarian to discuss any findings and have our vet do his or her own examination, run tests, give any necessary vaccinations and let me know of any special needs my dog may have.

Check into veterinary insurance or have a "Plan B" (credit card or separate bank account) so that if my dog needs medical care, I will be able to provide it.

Sign-up for a DOG FIRST-AID & CPCR Class and have a DOG FIRST-AID KIT (see page 111) on hand, so that I can help my best friend before veterinary care is available.

Cut out table scraps (except for carrots, bananas, string beans and other pet-friendly human foods) and keep my dog well exercised.

Brush my dog's teeth (or wipe the teeth and gums) at least every other day to prevent bacteria from travelling through my dog's bloodstream. See page 46.

Make sure my dog has a microchip and identification on him at all times and keep him safely in a fenced yard (with proper supervision) or walk him on a leash.

Enroll my dog in an obedience class (or give him a refresher on my own) so that he will be a welcome friend wherever we go together.

Provide my dog with a comfortable place to sleep in a warm, draft-free area.

Give my dog at least as much unconditional love as he gives me and spend good quality time with him for that is the greatest joy of being a Dog Parent!!!

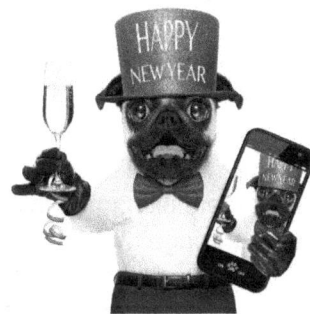

VALENTINE'S DAY

Life is Like a Box of Chocolates...Unless You Are a Dog!

The pathetic begging began and "the look" melted Milly's heart as she savored her Valentine chocolates with her Sheltie Duchess looking on. For this loving pet mom, resisting those big brown puppy dog eyes and telling her furry angel "No" grew increasingly more difficult as Duchess whimpered and whined, licking her tiny lips and cocking her head in the cutest way possible. Wanting what was best for her pooch, Milly created a diversion by putting away the chocolates, and then taking Duchess for a car ride (safely strapped in her doggie seat belt) to the local pet bakery for some dog-friendly treats. Not only did Milly know that once a dog tastes chocolate, she will want more (well, who doesn't?), but Milly was also aware that the sweet treat loved by humans everywhere can be deadly to our pets.

A study published in the 2006 Journal of Agricultural and Food Chemistry determined that chocolate is the third highest antioxidant source consumed in the U.S. following coffee and tea. According to Mark Stibich, PhD, "Chocolate is made from plants, which means it contains many of the health benefits of dark vegetables. These benefits are from flavonoids, which act as antioxidants which protect the body from aging caused by free radicals, which can cause damage that leads to heart disease. Dark chocolate contains a large number of antioxidants (nearly 8 times the number found in strawberries), and flavonoids help relax blood pressure and keep cholesterol from gathering in blood vessels."

Sounds good so far, but the benefits do not apply to the canine species! According to the ASPCA, its Animal Poison Control Center hotline receives an increased volume of calls from worried pet parents around Halloween, Christmas, Valentine's Day, Easter and Mother's Day, all holidays where candy is abundant. The problem isn't just the fat chocolate contains, but even worse, the caffeine-like substance known as theobromine a naturally occurring stimulant found in the cocoa bean. An animal that has ingested too much chocolate can experience rapid heart rate, vomiting, diarrhea, seizures and death. The only good news is that it takes a fairly large amount of Theobromine to cause a toxic reaction in your pet. However, do realize that every dog is different and some are much more sensitive to toxins than others meaning they can suffer ill effects on even the smallest amount of a substance.

So how much is too much chocolate for your dog? The darker the chocolate, the more dangerous for your pooch! White chocolate causes the least harm since it contains almost no cocoa and only 1mg of Theobromine per ounce. Milk chocolate, the most common form, contains 60mg per ounce which means: one ounce of milk chocolate per pound of your dog's body weight can be toxic! For example: 1/2 pound for an 8 lbs. dog or 4 pounds consumed by a 65 lbs. dog would make him very ill or worse. The chocolate generally found in chocolate chip cookies, semi-sweet chocolate, contains an even higher Theobromine concentration, so less than one ounce per pound your pet weighs can make him just as sick. Theobromine is found in still higher levels in dark chocolate, cocoa powder and bakers' chocolate as well as cocoa mulch which often adorns potted plants and flower beds.

Once swallowed, there is no specific antidote for chocolate poisoning, so if you suspect your dog has consumed chocolate, induce vomiting at once by administering one tablespoon of 3% hydrogen peroxide for every 15 lbs. your pet weighs. Dribble it onto the back of his tongue with an eye dropper, needle-less syringe or even a turkey baster until he swallows. As an alternative, activated charcoal may help absorb the toxins in your pet's stomach and buy you time to get to the animal emergency Center before the poison travels through your pet's bloodstream. Once at the Animal ER, the Veterinarian will flush your pet's system, give intravenous medications to protect his heart and treat whatever symptoms occur. So like Forrest Gump always said, "Life is like a box of chocolates. You never know what you're going to get." And for your dog or cat...it will never be a good thing, so NO CHOCOLATE FOR FIDO! Also, since you never know what unexpected events will be thrown your way, be prepared by having a well-stocked pet first-aid kit (page 111) along with the knowledge of what to do to help your pet in any kind of emergency.

Fourth of July Fireworks

The weeks before and after the Fourth of July are among the busiest at animal shelters across the country. Shelters fill up with strays often making staff have to choose which other animals must be euthanized to make room for the sudden influx. Loud booms and flashing fireworks make humans "oooooo" and "awwww", but they chase our dogs from the safety of their homes (not to mention the harm they bring to birds and other wildlife). Escaped dogs become disoriented and end up miles away from those who love them, and those are the lucky dogs who get picked up and taken to shelters. Many more meet their fate by running frantically into the path of a car.

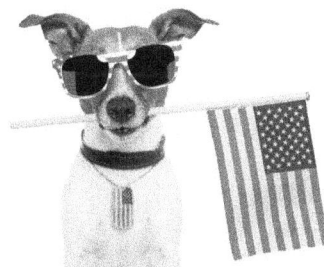

Be a responsible dog parent making sure to provide a safe environment for your four-legged best friends. Although you may be tempted to bring them along to enjoy the festivities, think again, and follow a few rules so that your dog will be safe and happy when the fifth of July rolls around.

Indoors

Close the drapes and turn on a radio or television to mask any noise and distract the dog's attention from the pops and bangs. Triple check that all doors, windows and gates are secure, and if your dog is easily agitated, make sure someone stays with him during the festivities.

Outdoors

Enjoy your cookout, but keep your dogs on their normal diet. Burgers, fries, salty chips, and fried chicken can all upset your pet's stomach while fats from an abundance of these foods can result in pancreatitis. Alcoholic beverages can result in a coma or respiratory failure. Chocolate can be lethal.

If swimming is on the agenda, make sure you watch Fido. Just because he's a dog doesn't mean he knows how to swim. For boating activities or when near lakes and streams, a doggie life-vest is appropriate attire.

Keep pets far away from sparklers and firecrackers. One spark on precious fur and you'll need an emergency trip to the Veterinarian. Do not let paw, snout or any part of your furry friend get close as the results could be deadly.

Back-to-School Tips

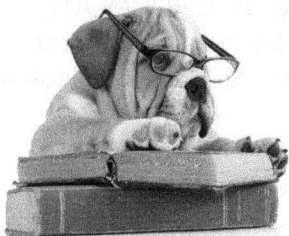

Things to keep in mind that can help the animals in your household adjust and stay safe:

When the school bell rings, don't let your dog go back to school too. A lonely pet may want to tag along. Keep your pet confined when children leave for school, and if you drive, don't take the dogs with you. Animals learn quickly and may find their own way to school later on resulting in them becoming lost or injured. For severe separation anxiety, place the t-shirt your child slept in the night before in your dog's bed -- as long as he doesn't rip it to shreds, it will make him feel like his boy or girl is there with him.

Now that mom or dad may be experiencing a little "empty nesting," it's a great time to spend extra quality time with the family pet. Embark on an exercise and training program for your dog. A tired dog is a good dog who will wait patiently for his "kids" to come home from school. Love and attention is a bow wow wonderful thing, but you don't want your dog to become a "velcro" pet sticking to your side every second of the day. Interest your dog in toys filled with treats in between training sessions and belly rubs. Just be careful though not to over-treat your pets and have them pack on the pounds.

Dogs are part of the family too, so make sure you focus extra attention on them when their world has suddenly been turned upside down by their humans' change of schedule.

Halloween

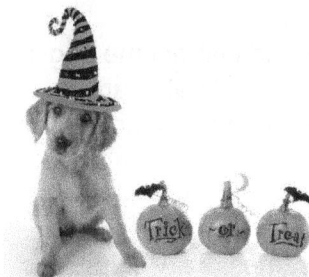

Things that go bump in the night shouldn't include your pets, so follow a few simple tips to make sure Howl-o-ween won't be scary or dangerous for canines!

PREVENT A HOUDINI ACT by knowing where your dogs are at all times. Walk them before dark and do not take them trick or treating. Many dogs get scared by the shrieks of ghosts & goblins on the streets or coming to their doors and they dart into the path of cars. Others are scared by masked and caped individuals moving towards them. Keep your dog in a quiet back room or on a leash safely at your side if you are answering the door to trick or treaters.

AVOID THE KISS OF DEATH from items ingested. Candy wrappers can cause intestinal blockages and chocolate can be fatal to dogs. If you're putting out creepy treats with grapes or raisins masquerading as "eyeballs," make sure your dogs do not get them as they can cause kidney failure. Keep plastic toothpicks that adorn festive cupcakes also out of reach, and take care that your dogs can't chew or become entangled in wires or electric cords. Ensure dogs steer clear of candles haunting the family jack o'lantern as well as fake spider webs and spray string, all of which can burn, choke or cause harm if ingested.

IF YOUR PET LOOKS MISERABLE...HE PROBABLY IS! Unless Fluffy is truly comfortable in a costume, their own furry birthday suit might be a better choice. A festive bandana on your dog might just fit the bill. Pets aren't used to wearing elastic and definitely don't like masks covering their eyes or nose, so think of your four-legged friend. Is that photo op worth them being uncomfortable? Should you have a dog willing to "dress up," make sure the costume doesn't have beads or strings which they may chew on, and never leave your dog unattended in a costume!

EVIL LURKS IN THE NIGHT, and some people, taking advantage of the anonymity of costumes, partake in malicious pranks targeting black cats, dogs and other animals. Even if you don't normally do so, please, please, please keep your dogs in the house on Halloween night. If you see anything suspicious regarding the treatment of an animal, immediately call your local animal control or police department. See if your city has its own animal cruelty task force.

And remember...September and October can still be very HOT in some locations! Make sure your dogs have plenty of shade and water. Never leave them unattended in a parked car and be certain that kennels, pet carriers and even rooms in your house are cool with good ventilation for your pooch.

Thanksgiving

Giving your dog a small nibble of white-meat turkey is okay, just be sure it's boneless and fully cooked. Bones can splinter and dark meat, greasy skin, gristle and gravies can cause severe stomach upsets and pancreatitis in your four-legged friends for which there is no cure! The inflammation to the pancreas (the organ responsible for insulin and enzyme production vital to digestion) must resolve on its own during a period of hospitalization, administration of IV fluids, medication and round-the-clock monitoring for life-threatening complications.

Sweet potato, cooked carrots and green beans — inside a stuffed toy — will keep canines delighted and too busy to come begging for table scraps. Pumpkin puree, although beneficial to a pet suffering from fur balls, constipation or diarrhea, can cause concern if ingested in the form of pumpkin pie or pie mix due to the added sugar, spices and other ingredients. Also, don't overdue pumpkin, as it is a remedy for constipation and too much can give your pet the runs.

Although sage makes stuffing taste yummy, it contains essential oils and resins that can cause pets to suffer stomach upset and possible depression of the central nervous system, so be sure to keep this herb out of reach.

If you're letting yeast dough rise on the counter, make sure Fido don't come near. Raw dough in a canine tummy continues to ferment and can result in alcohol poisoning!

Family gatherings bring relatives and friends who may not be as pet savvy as you! Politely give guests a few rules about closing doors and gates behind them so that your precious dogs do not escape. Provide a safe place for toothpicks that may be used with hors d'oeuvres, as once dropped on the floor with the aroma of meats and cheeses, these sharp objects become desirable to our pets and can cause puncture and choking injuries.

Be sure to safely tuck away bones, foils and plastic wraps from your pets. The food remnants on these items will make them hard to resist and could cause obstructions, choking incidents and even suffocation to your pet.

The holiday season means lots of cameras, radios and other battery-operated electronics. Please don't leave batteries lying around. If swallowed, they can cause choking or obstruction; if punctured, the chemicals in alkaline batteries can cause burns to the mouth and esophagus.

Finally, holidays often translate to candies and sweets. Read Chocolate Toxicity on page 74, but also realize the wrappers and artificial sweeteners in some treats can be extremely harmful to our pets. Nuts are hard for pets to digest and some, such as macadamia, can cause temporary paralysis. Just because people eat it DOES NOT mean it is safe for our dogs.

Count your blessings during this season of thanks and be ever so grateful that a four-legged friend has chosen to share his life with you!!!

Christmas / Hannukah / Kwanzaa & Other Festive Celebrations

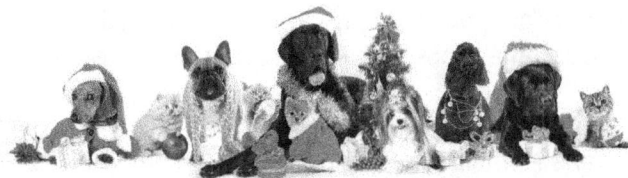

Put yourself in your dog's paws… At the end of each year, boxes are dragged from the garage or attic and unusual things happen in their home. A tree is brought INDOORS; shiny, dangly things are hung all around, and there's always food on the counter or baking in the oven while people come in and out shouting greetings!

As you decorate, whether it be electric cords, candles, pine trees or ribbon, realize any of these can be problematic and that your pet should never be allowed to explore around them without supervision. ***Don't block pathways with decorations.*** If your dog watches the mailman every day from a certain window in your home, DO NOT put the Christmas tree or candle display in that window!

Make sure your puppy or dog has a **safe refuge** when company comes, music gets too loud or there is any type of commotion so that they can feel safe. Also provide them with something in a quiet place to keep them out of mischief — safe toys and maybe even quietly play music or a radio to drown out noise coming from the boisterous humans.

Giving pets as gifts is a very bad idea! People and families should choose the dog that is right for them, one who fits into their lifestyle and at a time they are capable of giving it a forever home. If however you have decided to adopt a dog for yourself at this time of year, that is a wonderful thing! Remember baby dogs are like baby humans in that they need extra care and constant watching. They have not learned any of life's rules yet or the methods for their own survival, so…Don't upset their routine. Keep feeding and playtimes on schedule in spite of company or other obligations, and don't delay in cleaning up or walking the dog in spite of your extra busy schedule.

When choosing to adopt a dog during the holidays, you should consider whether or not you are willing to take a "time out" from the season. We're not saying you can't enjoy festivities because sharing them with your new best friend can be awesome, but a new dog needs time to transition into his new life and can't do so if you are dashing about, stressed, or have a constant stream of company coming and going. It's important for you to get off on the right paw and let your new furry family member know that this is now their home too and that you are their special person and will always be there for them. Remember, dogs need many outside breaks and time with you to run off their energy. If you've answered yes to all of these basic pet parenting obligations and agree to the commitment, then by all means, adopt as dogs need homes for the holidays and shouldn't have to wait in a shelter a moment longer than necessary. But waiting for their soul mate person is better than being adopted into a home and lifestyle that is not ready for them. When humans get too overwhelmed, pets feel our frustration and often get returned to shelters, so make sure you are ready, and that is the best time to adopt!

Although poinsettias are the first **plants** that come to mind as a hazard around pets, they are not as dangerous as others, usually only erupting into digestive upsets. Holly, mistletoe, pine cones and pine needles can cause problems ranging from obstructions, intestinal perforations to vomiting, diarrhea and lethargy. Poisoning is relative depending on the amount of poison ingested vs. the size of the dog. See Poisonous Plant Chart on page 234. Make sure dogs do not drink water from live Christmas trees as the sap, as well as any water additives, can be problematic. Cut an X in a plastic lid that will fit over the water reservoir or cover with foil. Placing "sticky tape" around your tree skirt or anything with a bumpy surface (such as an upside down floor or car mat that have those nubs dogs won't like to step on) may make your dog take a step back.

Ribbons, bows, yarn and tinsel as well as cranberry and popcorn garlands on your tree or packages can entice any pet. The strings not only can cause choking and blockages but can also wrap around your dog's tongue while the other end gets pulled by intestinal contractions.

Homemade ornaments and play dough made from salt and flour can be lethal if ingested. Boxes and paper bags are generally a safe play toy for your furry friends but just be extra safe in checking these items before you toss them as kitty could be hanging out in one!

Hanging dog biscuits on the branches however is just asking for trouble. As a precaution, secure your tree to a wall or a cup hook in the ceiling with pretty ribbon or invisible fishing wire so that at the least, it won't fall if your pup goes for a climb. Placing a decorative child gate (think pretty white pickets) around the base may prevent your pup from getting too near and keep them safe through the season.

As for holiday eats... A little boiled or broiled white meat chicken or turkey is usually not a bad idea, although you may be surprised to learn that more and more dogs have allergies to chicken, beef and even fish! The key is moderation and staying away from dark meats, cooked fats and skins, gravies and anything slathered with oils, butter or salt. If you slip a little turkey into your dog's bowl it's one thing, but remind Uncle Bob, Cousin Charlie, Grandma, your sister- in-law and the kid down the street not to also do the same. Pancreatitis can result which means your pet will need to spend the holidays in intensive care at your local Animal ER! Dogs can metabolize fat, bone, and gristle from animals caught in the wild but once we cook fat it becomes grease; cooked bones splinter, so stick to their appropriate diet and give them safe treats. Watch out for the dropped rum balls and brandy soaked cakes as well. Cooked carrot slices, broccoli or string beans (without the salt and butter) can be a nice change; dehydrate liver or fish or make another dog treat yourself so that you know what is in it.

When keeping food hot during parties, make sure Sterno™-type canisters remain out of paws reach. They may look like pet food, and although considered "green" and clean burning, they contain ethanol and methanol which are toxic if ingested by your dog!

Don't let pets lick up spills or lick out of wine or cocktail glasses. A small amount of alcohol for a small creature can result in serious symptoms. Grapes or raisins, chocolate or caffeine products all pose dangers to our feline friends as do nuts and too much dairy (including cheeses). So supervise bowls of nuts and candies — especially if the candies are in wrappers and the cellophane too could be consumed.

Dedicate playtime just for you and your dog(s) BEFORE company arrives, and then let the dogs retreat to a quiet back bedroom with safe toys of their own to play with. Know how your dog reacts to people and noise. Welcome your pooch to join and if you feel they can make a brief appearance, but remind children not to bother dogs while they are eating and not to pull the ears or tail.

TRAVEL SAFETY

Every year thousands of animals are injured, die or become lost in car accidents. They can be thrown against dashboards, windows, seat backs or floors.

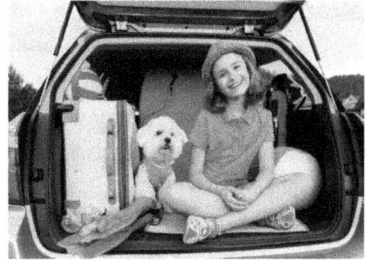

"Wearing your seat belt costs you nothing," states Nicole Nason of the National Highway Traffic Safety Administration (NHTSA), "but the cost for not wearing one certainly will." This applies to pets too! A 50 pound dog traveling 30 mph will feel like nine 170 pound men pushed him against a brick wall if he is thrown during an accident (that's "ruff"ly 1,500 lbs. of force!) Unrestrained pets who survive may still suffer devastating injuries. Others escape the car through broken windows and now-open doors only to end up being struck by on-coming vehicles.

Cause of Accidents
Pets are often the cause of accidents. According to the American Automobile Association (AAA), animals moving around in cars are the third worst distraction to a driver ranking only behind children and cell phones.

Ways to Keep Your Pets Safe
No excuses! Buckle Fido into a special pet seatbelt even if it's only a ride around the block. Dog restraints easily attach to your vehicle's seat belt and allow your pet to sit up or lie down. Many varieties can be purchased at pet stores and on-line. Wire cages or plastic crates are also good choices as they shield dogs from falling objects. Just make sure the crate too is secured so that it along with your dog does not become a projectile during an impact or sudden stop.

Do Not Let Your Dog Ride With His Head Out the Window

Gravel, tree branches, dust, pollen and even the breeze may result in infection, injury or trauma to his eyes. If his head is out the window and his paw steps on a power button, the window could close on his neck!

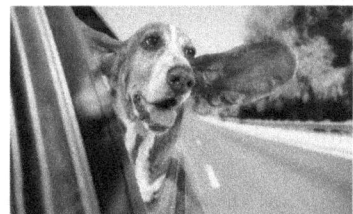

Do not Let Your Dog Ride "Shotgun"
If the airbag is deployed it could crush a small pet or break his neck. Even inside a fiberglass crate, it is not safe for a pet to ride in the front seat! Airbags often result in larger dogs severing the lingual artery in their tongues from the force of their teeth slamming together. This would place your dog in an emergency situation incurring heavy blood loss and it is likely that if the airbag has been deployed neither you nor your car will be capable of transporting your injured pet.

Never Let Your Dog Ride Unrestrained in the Bed of a Pick-up Truck

Many cities now prohibit this practice altogether while others are considering laws to make pet restraint mandatory in all vehicles. If truck bed transport is absolutely necessary, be double doggone sure that:

1) The space is enclosed or has side and tail racks to a height of no less than 46 inches extending vertically from the bed.
2) The dog is cross-tethered to the vehicle using a harness that encircles his shoulders and rib cage (Never attach tethering or leashes to a neck collar in a moving vehicle!).
3) Your pet is protected by a secured container or cage that cannot fall or slide about.

Several campaigns have been launched to help you become proactive for the safety of your pet, and new products become available all the time, so become a savvy pet parent keeping your eyes open for new ways to keep your best friend safe.

When going out of town, have your pet examined by your Veterinarian and make sure vaccinations are current. Next, get your dog acclimated to the car by taking short trips close to home. Should your traveling companion need a bit of calming, CDs are available that can relax the whole family en route as can aromatherapy sprays that spritz anxiety away. Vicki Rae Thorne of Earth Heart, LLC who has been blending essential oils for 20 years suggests, "Lavender, tangerine and rose geranium can have a calming effect while bergamot has been used for anxiety and ginger for stomach upset. "Toys as well as frequent walks are a must, and NEVER leave your dog alone in the car for even a few minutes. Despite windows rolled down, cars get very hot very fast and your best friend could suffer brain damage.

Choosing Your Mode of Transportation

Cars & Similar Vehicles
Once buckled in safely, enjoy the journey! According to the Travel Industry Association of America more than 29 million Americans have traveled with their pets over the last several years spending $28 million on travel in 2012 alone! Jim Simmons and his dog Darby are no exception. They have ridden aboard a 1938 restored antique fire engine, on a horse drawn wagon and even a pontoon boat. Simmons documented their adventures in the travel show "Across Indiana," and father and dog continue to create wonderful memories together.

Host of PBS' "Animal Attractions TV" Megan Blake loves traveling by car with her dogs. "I can reach over and pet them anytime, and in Los Angeles traffic, a dog pet can be a great stress reliever! I also have more control in my own car. We are not subject to flight delays or schedule changes, and the sight-seeing is great!"

Laurie Lee Dovey of Pennsylvania feels, "Recreational vehicles are the only way to go." One thing she suggests you bring along is outdoor fencing which allows you to set up a perimeter for you and your pets at the campground.

Although not all canines were born to be easy riders, Emma Zen, a rescued Labrador-Great Dane is the exception. She has logged over 40,000 miles in her specially equipped Harley Davidson Sidecar, and makes an annual trek from California to Sturgis, South Dakota creating awareness about pet oxygen masks – many fire departments are now equipped with these animal life-saving devices thanks to the Emma Zen Foundation. When asked, "Why do you make your dog do that?" Emma's mom Debra Jo Chiapuzio smiles and says, "She loves it. It's her thing. You can see the joy in her face." In response to safety, Debra Jo explains, "Emma is harnessed to the seat from both sides. She wears eye protection, has sunscreen on her nose and ears and wears a T-shirt to keep the sun off, or a jacket when it's cold. We stop every hour and make Emma get out, move her body and be a dog." Debra Jo is trained in Pet First-Aid & CPR and has helped many animals, but always has her eyes wide open to keep Emma safe and cautions that the thrill of the wind whipping through your fur can be exhilarating, but it is not for every dog. So…unless you are a seasoned biker like Emma Zen who has parents like Debra Jo and Jim who go the extra mile to keep you safe, stick to an enclosed vehicle.

TIPS FOR DECREASING MOTION SICKNESS:

1) Allow your dog to spend good quality time in the car with you without the engine running and give him positive reinforcement for good behavior.
2) Follow this up with short trips around the block slowly building up to a fun nearby destination such as a park or trip through a drive through.

NOTE: A couple ginger snap cookies 20 minutes before any car ride often settles some queasy canine tummies. If using pure ginger capsules, give 100 mg per 25 lbs. of body weight 30 minutes before departure and repeat every 8 hours.

Aromatherapy sprays take effect more quickly than ingested herbs and can be applied within minutes of departure. The mist can be massaged onto the outer ears or abdomen of the pet or sprayed on his favorite blanket.

3) As you increase road travel, always make sure it is on an empty stomach – that your pet has not eaten for 4-6 hours.
4) Confining your dog not only makes safety sense, but it restricts his movement lessening the likelihood of nausea. If your pup is riding in a crate or carrier, facing the crate forward helps prevent motion sickness. If you must turn it in another direction for safety sake, cover it to prevent your pet looking out in a non-forward moving direction. For safely restraining a pet while traveling (see page 81).
5) If you have more than one vehicle, try them out with Rover. Some cars vibrate more or are more conducive to motion sickness than others.
6) Keep the car cool inside.

7) If motion sickness seems to be an ongoing problem for your dog, speak to your Veterinarian about Cerenia (maropitant citrate) or other prescription medications that won't make him drowsy but will allow him to spend his time on four wheels with you. As with all drugs, follow directions to the letter for your pet's sake.

8) If the problem seems more anxiety related, aromatherapy with lavender may prove beneficial in keeping nerves at bay.

Planes

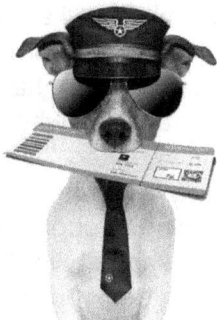

If you need to get there fast, a plane may be your choice of transport. Check with the various commercial carriers for their rules and regulations to see which can best accommodate your dog on board. Air Hollywood's K9 Flight School prepares people and pets to travel confidently and comfortably by providing valuable information and training in an immersive aviation environment. It might be good to give this a try before emBARKing on the real thing!

If your dog must ride in the cargo hold, here are some considerations to increase the chances of a safe flight:

• Familiarize him with his travel carrier weeks before the flight and don't forget a pre-travel veterinary visit.
• Clip nails so that they can't catch on carrier doors, and make sure the collar also cannot catch on anything.
• Don't feed for 4-6 hours prior to air travel. Place ice cubes in the tray attached to the inside of the crate. Water will spill.
• Once through security it will be hours before a potty break, so exercise before hand.
• Book only direct flights and chose early morning/late evening flights during the hot months and afternoon flights during the colder times of year. Avoid holiday chaos at all costs for your pet's sake.
• Travel on the same flight and watch your dog being loaded and unloaded.
• Let the captain and flight attendants know your dog is traveling in the cargo hold.
• Label the carrier with your name, permanent address and telephone number, final destination, and where you or a contact person can be reached as soon as the flight arrives.
• Upon arrival, open the carrier as soon as you are in a safe place and if anything appears not quite right, high tail it to a Veterinarian.

The Humane Society warns that riding underneath a plane could expose animals to temperature extremes, poor ventilation and rough handling. Unless your Veterinarian advises differently, NEVER fly flat-snouted dogs including Pugs, Pekingese and Chow Chows in the cargo hold. These breeds have short nasal passages that leave them vulnerable to oxygen deprivation and heat stroke.

Trains

Traveling by train may be considered a cultural experience, but canines don't get it, and the noise and vibration may be a stressful experience. Most dogs must ride in cargo without climate controls, so consider the time of year and all the usual travel precautions such as ID-ing your pet, acclimating him ahead of time, how frequently you can exercise him and everything else you can think of to make his journey stress-free.

Boats and Ships

On the water make sure your dog wears a life vest at all times – no matter how good of a swimmer he is! Most have a handle on top the dog's back that assists you in lifting him out of the water in an emergency. With four paws on a wet deck, fiberglass can be challenging, so provide a rubber mat to help paws take hold and to protect from hot surfaces.

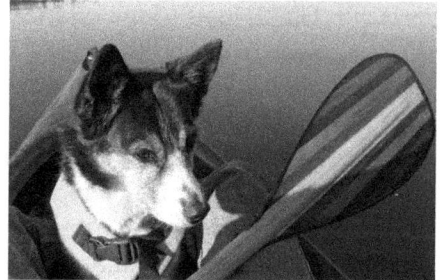

Author, TV host and creator of dogfessions.com Nikki Moustaki traveled aboard the Queen Mary II with her Schnauzer Pepper in celebration of ten years together. It took eight months of preparation, but it was all worthwhile. On board the ship, the dogs stay in a kennel area, which has a deck run with a spectacular view where they get plenty of exercise and a playroom as well as the room with cages. According to Nikki, "The dogs are out of the cages pretty much all day and have free run of these areas. Cunard has generous visiting hours all day long." Nikki advises that, "If you are confused about anything, call the carrier!" You don't want any surprises once you're ready to board.

Where to Stay & What to Do

According to Kelley E. Carter, author of National Geographic's The Dog Lover's Guide to Travel, "The travel industry, realizing that you consider Fido a full-fledged family member, has changed with the times. Hotels that don't accept hounds are passe, and many upscale hotels have taken dog friendly to new heights."

Yet do your homework! Some locales only allow dogs up to a certain weight, others require dogs to be kenneled when you aren't there and others just don't have anything for dogs to do. If you don't have time for all the research on your own, Pet Friendly Accommodations Worldwide (PAW) or Furlocity can be your one stop shop. PAW President Janine Francheschi and her Irish Setter Beau have driven 20,000 miles, visited 30 states and stayed in hundreds of three-star or higher hotels. They rate locales on being not just 'pet-accepting' but genuinely 'pet-friendly,' says Janine. "Dining in these cities with your pet is easy because of the abundance of sidewalk cafe's and outdoor dining venues." The Furlocity team are also pet parents themselves who rid you of the cumbersome and outdated process and offer first class web technology to find and book your next stay for you and your pooch.

Must-Haves for the Traveling Canine: Your Dog's Travel Kit

No matter where you go, there are items Fido should not be without:

- Health certificate/vaccination records in duplicate
- Medications and supplements (flea & tick prevention)
- Bowls (food and water)
- Usual food (don't chance a stomach upset by switching on the road)
- Water (in the car and plane, ice cubes work best when available)
- Treats and/or Meal Replacement Bars
- Micro-chip and ID tag on a securely fitting collar
- Extra leashes, harness, seat belt
- Dog First-Aid Kit and handbook
- Ginger snaps to settle an upset tummy
- Canned or dehydrated pumpkin puree (no added ingredients unless plain apple fiber) for most kinds of digestive upsets (vomiting, diarrhea and constipation)
- Information regarding Veterinarians and 24 Hour Pet Emergency Hospitals (a great resource is "Pet E.R. Guide" by Melinda Lord, Trailer Life Books but also check for up-to-date Apps)
- Bedding and something that smells like home
- Toys
- Crate
- Dog brush & towels
- Lint brushes or packaging tape so you don't leave too much hair wherever you go
- Dog shoes for snow or rough terrain

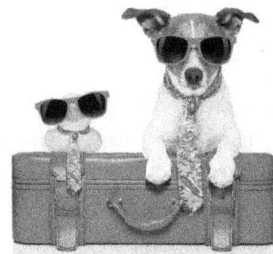

Pet Travel Expert Janine Franceschi says , "The most important item I carry when Beau and I travel together is a complete copy of all of his medical records. You hope you never need them, but when you do it makes life so much easier to have them handy than trying to get in touch with a vet thousands of miles away."

Not all dogs have this luxury, but one thing Pamela Biery never forgets is her Pug's Therapy Vest. This obviously only applies to true service dogs. "Not only does it allow him to go into places where he otherwise would not be able to go, but it is critical during the summer since it's not safe to leave pets in cars in even fairly mild weather." Sherlock McBiskit, a Westie from Charlotte, NC never travels without his beanie babies. Bobbi Leder and her English Cocker remind that a waterproof liner is an asset in the car or anywhere, and Debra Jo Chiapuzio recommends that you also "bring along knowledge and peace of mind by knowing what to do in an emergency situation – learn pet first-aid and CPR." See Section II of this book to get yourself up-to-speed on these skills.

Disaster Preparedness

Do your research now and gather your tools, so that if an emergency occurs, you can turn tragedy into a success story for your four-legged family members.

Hopefully you will never experience a fire destroying your home, yet you plan ahead -- install fire alarms, smoke detectors and purchase insurance. You certainly hope never to be involved in a car accident, but you have airbags and wear a seat belt (and should safely restrain your dog as well). Being prepared makes sense as we can minimize potential injury to those we love. However, most people are not prepared for a major disaster. "Be Prepared" works for the Scouts, and it's a motto we should carry into our adult lives. Planning ahead is the best way to keep yourself and your dog safe.

At The Very Least:

1) Place a Pet Alert Sticker near you front door recording how many and what type of animals live there. If you aren't home when tragedy strikes, trained professionals will seek out and help your pets.

Photo: Sunny-dog Ink

2) Designate a pre-arranged meeting place for your family and identify several places that can take your pets. Red Cross Shelters do not permit pets. Many organizations train communities to set-up temporary animal shelters, but it could still be days before these facilities are in place. Making arrangements ahead of time with out-of-town friends and relatives is your best bet, but have a "Plan B." Susan Keyes, President of the Southern California Animal Response Team says, "Long-term housing and care for pets is the area we have found people to be least prepared." Check with pet day care and boarding facilities as well as your Veterinarian to see if they will accommodate during a disaster. Compile a list of hotels where pets are welcome and set aside one credit card just for emergency use. It's also a good idea to have cash (in bills smaller than 20s) easily accessible as ATM Machines will not be working.

Know Dog-friendly (and learn what that means, ie: breeds, weight and size may play a role) locations before you need them. Publisher Susan Sims and her team at "Fido Friendly" are a great place to start your research.

3) Stash the following for each pet in an easy-to-carry backpack or crate (that way you'll have the carrier to evacuate in):
   • A two-week supply of food stored in an airtight container and a manual can opener if needed; water (for medium to large dogs, one gallon per day); medication. Remember to exchange these items regularly so they are fresh when needed.

- A water-proof container with vaccination & micro-chipping records and photos of your pet with your family as proof of ownership.
- Treats, toys, bedding, food & water dishes; collars/harnesses and leashes; disinfectant for cleaning crates, paper towels, flashlight with batteries, zip ties, garbage bags and a well-stocked Pet First-Aid Kit.

4) Stay Informed by listening to media announcements for frequent updates. As the saying goes, "Knowledge is power," so don't be caught unaware.

See Pet Disaster Pawparedness Checklist on page 230.

Where To Put It All

Even with the best laid plans, life happens, so consider storing your goods in several locations in the event they are un-retrievable when the ground shakes, the flames rise or the mud slides. Positioning items close to an outside wall in your home will allow easier access should buildings collapse and you need to rummage through rubble to get to your supplies. Also, stowing duplicate items in your car is a good idea.

Don't Forget The Two-Legged Family Members

Also remember to keep a stash of food and other items for the humans including a battery or solar-powered radio, rubber-soled shoes and a flashlight near your bed so that you can help your pets and stay safe!

Determine well in advance which rooms are safest should you need to hunker down (center of house, bathrooms, closets, basements, or other room depending on type of impending danger.)

In situations where water supply may become contaminated, fill up bathtubs and sinks to ensure that you have access to water during a power outage or other crises.

Preparing for the worst may just prevent the worst from happening!

Tips for Specific Disasters

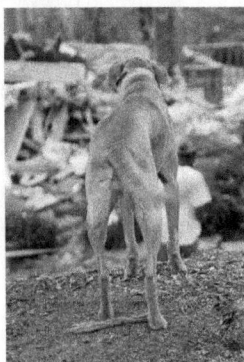

Although it is difficult to teach someone not to get stressed, being as prepared as you can be for any situation in life can help lessen the panic that sets in when the worst happens.

Follow general disaster preparedness Tips, but also take special care depending on which of the following natural disasters are likely to occur in your part of the world.

Hurricanes

The one good thing to be said about hurricanes is that they are predictable -- The National Hurricane Center tracks weather patterns and notes possible disturbances long before they pose a threat. It's imperative that you monitor your local news channels and once a Hurricane Watch is issued, although you may have 24 - 36 hours before it hits, don't wait to do the following:

- Keep dogs indoors and easily accessible should you need to suddenly pack them up and leave.
- Stay tuned to news stations for evacuation routes and make sure you completely understand the plan.
- Have at least one week's food, water and any medications stored for your dogs and prep your house for the storm (board-up windows, stow away items that can blow such as patio furniture, secure gates, etc.).

A Hurricane Warning is issued when the storm is 24 hours away or less. Complete all preparations before the rain and high winds arrive, and stay in your home only if it is safe. If you evacuate, take Fido and Fluffy with you.

Wildfires

Once underway, wildfires can consume millions of acres and blow in changing directions. For this reason, you should plan several escape routes for you and your dogs in the event the flames block your path.

- Create a "fire break" around your home by clearing away vegetation, especially dead brush, about 30 feet from all structures.
- Use fabric, rope or leather leashes and collars. Nylon ones melt when heated and can badly burn your pooch.
- Take all animals with you. Monitor your pets for burns and smoke inhalation. Knowing how to perform Rescue Breathing & CPR could save your dog's life!

Earthquakes

Unlike most natural disasters, there is no advanced warning for an earthquake allowing no time for last minute precautions. In addition to covering the steps above:

- Never position dog runs, crates or enclosures underneath objects that could fall during a tremor.
- Add a pair of bolt cutters to your disaster kit in case damaged cages or fencing need opening.
- Know where to turn off the gas to your house, barn or kennels.
- Include your dogs in the family earthquake drill and make sure all family members know how to handle them realizing that a frightened dog may bite or scratch.
- If you board your dog, make sure the facility knows of your earthquake preparedness plans.

Should an earthquake occur, confine your pets. Dogs that escape sometimes return at mealtime, but there are no guarantees! Be prepared to handle cut and burned paws, know how to splint broken bones and stop bleeding in humans and animals alike. In other words, take a Dog First-Aid Class before you wish you had.

Floods

Floods can affect any part of the world and can even be confined to only your home or apartment building. Every year hundreds of thousands of people are forced to evacuate due to rising water. Slowly rising water is usually due to rivers, streams or even a pipe leak in your home. Flash floods however can hit quickly caused by heavy rain or melting snow as well as failure to a dam or reservoir.

- Map out several evacuation routes for yourself and your four-legged family; don't rely on only one which may be in the path of the floodwater. Head for the nearest high ground with your pets, and it is always better to err on the side of caution and evacuate early. If it is a false alarm, you and your family have practiced a meaningful drill instead of the real thing.
- Never leave any animal behind and certainly don't tie up an animal if flood waters threaten. You cannot anticipate how high water may rise, so even birds enclosed on high perches could perish.
- Remember that danger of disease can be an issue after a flood. Keep dogs away from standing water. Have a good fresh supply of water on hand for everyone (1/2 gallon per day for small dogs; 1 gallon for larger animals) as even tap water may not be safe if contaminated water has entered the drinking supply.

Make Your Older Dog's Years Golden

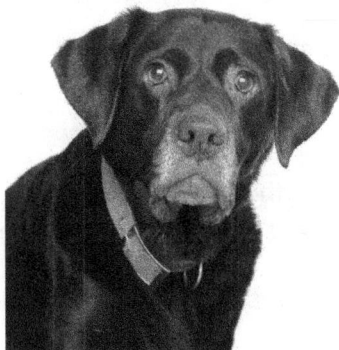

With the ceremonial lighting of candle #7 on the doggie bone birthday cake, it is generally assumed your best friend has embarked on his golden years. With larger breeds though, the elder years could arrive earlier. Though often premature to consider him a senior citizen, it's a great time to make changes that can ensure a continuing quality of life.

Decreased activity and loss of muscle tone can result in constipation, arthritis, degenerative joint disease and cognitive dysfunction, so get those paws moving. But always speak with your Veterinarian before starting any new regimen to be sure it is the best course of action for your pet and bring your pet in for a senior wellness exam.

Canines and humans experience many of the same aging patterns: graying hair, aches, pains and stiffness, sleeping more and slowing down. One big difference though is that our dogs can't tell us what hurts or what isn't working as good as it used to. Your Veterinarian can be a great source in determining your pet's needs, but you are even better. Pay attention, really get to know your dog and observe any changes to insure his later years will be truly golden.

Exercise helps maintain healthy body weight -
Just as in humans, excess weight in senior pets
may bring about serious health conditions. Without
proper exercise, the increased bulk stresses an
older dog's heart. When this organ doesn't function
properly, other organs like the brain, lungs, liver
and kidneys suffer too. Exercise also aids in proper
digestion and nutrient absorption which are important
to overall health.

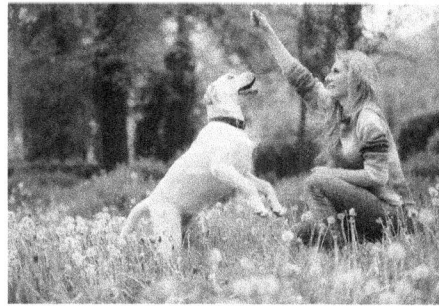

Exercise helps delay the onset of osteoarthritis – We all need our joints to work
smoothly and efficiently to get us where we want to go. Moderate exercise can keep
movement fluid, slow deterioration and minimize pain.

Exercise helps maintain mental health – Well-oxygenated blood flow to tissues does
a body good, and exercise also removes toxins. Activity keeps nutrients like glucose at
optimum levels in the brain and like every other organ in the body, the brain requires
good nutrition to function properly.

Quality time with and loving touch from you – It has been discovered that human touch
can stimulate parts of the brain that control emotions in human Alzheimer patients so why
not give it a try with your furry best friend?

What's a dog parent to do?
- First, talk to your Veterinarian to determine what exercises will be most beneficial
  and which to avoid.
- If at any time your dog gets tired, coughs or has problems breathing, stop and call
  your vet. You know your dog better than anyone else and know when he is not
  acting normal. By detecting and treating a problem early, you may save your best
  friend's life.
- Remain patient with your older dog and never get frustrated by time needed to
  acquire a new skill or perform a task. Enjoy each moment together.

What not to do:
- Do not let your senior canine exercise for long periods of time or under hot or
  humid conditions. Most dogs wish to please their owner and will risk their own
  health to do so.
- Do not force your senior to exercise. If he looks tired or unwilling, call a time-out.
  Limping, stiffness, lameness, tenderness in limbs and spinal areas are all reason
  to seek veterinary advice.
- Don't over-treat during training as older dogs add weight more quickly and lose
  pounds more slowly due to changes in their metabolism.

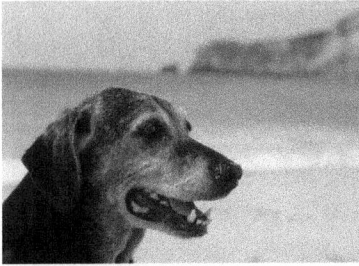

Studies show walking uphill may improve the flexibility of joints, particularly of the hip, while walking over low obstacles may improve the bending of a dog's joints in the front and rear limbs. Dogs who have undergone surgery to the tibia, however should avoid walking over obstacles which could potentially strain the tendon that joins the knee to the shin. Choosing the right exercise makes it beneficial as well as fun.

Speak with your dog's team of professionals to learn what is best for his particular situation.

Low impact walking and swimming are great ways to increase mobility. Short 10-15 minute sessions allow your dog to adjust to the routine without becoming tired. Aqua-therapy, with a combination of water resistance and free-joint movement, allows senior dogs to enjoy exercise with no harsh impact on their bodies.

If your dog however does not love to swim, choose another activity. Gentle walks during the cooler part of the day can be ideal. Build upon your dog's existing strengths and interests. One canine will be excellent at fetch and release, another might prefer tug-of-war, but the combination of mental and physical stimulation makes for the best workout.

As in any training or exercise program, pay attention to your dog and note if he is enjoying it. Break the activity into small achievable steps and reinforce the skill while encouraging progress. Consistency is vital for dogs that have lost an important communication tool such as sight or hearing. Use consistent commands or hand signals and be patient if your dog struggles to accommodate his new limitations.

Refresher courses on basic obedience keep an older mind sharp. Take your senior through his "sits," "stays" and "comes." Toss in something he never learned before whether it's that silly "keep the biscuit on your nose" trick or guessing which cup the kibble is under. Old dogs can learn new tricks. Be patient and keep it fun.

Nose work is also great for older dogs since it doesn't require physical stamina and can be enjoyed even by those losing their sight. It's a great way to keep the body busy and the mind active without over exerting. And agility isn't out of the question. Just slow down the speed and limit or leave out the jumps all together.

Whatever you do, do it together and cherish those golden years!

A Few PAWSitive Actions to Keep Your Senior Dog Comfy

1) Canines and humans experience many of the same aging patterns -- graying hair, aches, pains and stiffness, sleeping more and slowing down. One big difference though is that our ***pets can't tell us what hurts or what isn't working as good as it used to.*** Your veterinarian can be a great source in determining your pet's needs, but you are even better. Pay attention, really get to know your dog and observe any changes to insure his later years will be truly golden.

2) As animals age, <u>they often can't "hold it,"</u> and need more frequent bathroom breaks. Other times they have trouble remembering to ask to go out. <u>Don't lose patience</u> with your loyal companion. Instead, schedule extra outside breaks even if you have to come home at lunch or install a doggie door to a secure yard. Pick up water bowls two hours before bedtime and take pets out before you call it a night. Reduce clean-up by lining dog beds with plastic. Help your dog and help yourself by doing things that will make life easier.

3) All dogs should have <u>a special place of their own</u>, but senior pets should have <u>a bed in a draft- free, damp-free location</u> – something they can easily get out of but that cushions their aching joints. Observe your dog for his choice of location; some like the comfort of an egg-crate mattress while others prefer the coolness of the floor. Heavy-coated and short-nosed breeds need cooler temperatures while dogs with thin coats and arthritis need warmth.

4) <u>Elevating food and water bowls</u> may aid in digestion and prevent dogs from gulping excess air. It also lessens the strain on older bones by reducing how far they bend. Work with your veterinarian to find solutions for your breed.

5) <u>Supplements</u> - Talk with your veterinarian or holistic practitioner about other supplements that could help maintain healthy tendons, ligaments, joints and cartilage such as: Glucosamine Sulfate with MSM, Chondroitin Hyaluronic Acid and others. Other supplements may positively impact your dog's lifestyle including Vitamin E, Melatonin, Essential Fatty Acids and Curcumin for example, but check with your dog's medical professional. Don't just add these items to your dog's diet without knowing how they might react with other medications or treatments.

6) A dog with (or without) hearing loss must be protected by being <u>kept on-leash</u> when out of the house or yard. As senses dim, your pet won't hear approaching traffic, children or other animals coming near. When startled he may snap or bite out of fear. Be aware of changes. Teach everyone to gently stomp their feet to <u>create a vibration</u> your pet can feel and call out when approaching a hearing or vision impaired pet. <u>Use hand signals</u> when your voice can no longer be heard; flick kitchen lights to teach your deaf pet that it's time for dinner.

7) <u>Don't rearrange the furniture!</u> Dogs with fading sight memorize their pathways. Keep them safe by installing a gate near stairs so that they can't take a tumble, and build a wide, sturdy ramp over steps your dog frequents.

8) <u>Various modalities</u> such as chiropractic adjustments, massage (see page 29), stretching, aquatic therapy and acupuncture can make a world of difference in the mobility of some senior dogs.

9) If Fido cannot be on the go with you as much as in the past, <u>make time</u> for belly rubs and do whatever he can do…short walks, car rides or just being together. Senior pets do best when they know they are loved and are still a treasured part of the family.

End of Life Decisions

The loss of a beloved pet can be devastating as our dogs are part of our family. As your dog gets on in yours or develops a chronic condition, talk with the family about what is best for your best friend. Although wonderful advances in medicine, putting your pet through surgery and extensive medication may not provide them the best quality of life for their golden years. Although we selfishly may not want to say good bye, euthanasia administered by a caring veterinarian with your family present may be the kindest last gift you can give your dog. Investigate professionals who come to your home to make that transition easier as well as offer tips on how to make those last days, weeks and months memorable for all.

Before the time comes, decide on a pet cemetery or having your dog cremated. Most cities do not allow burying of pets in your backyard, so research ahead so you won't hit road blocks while you are grieving.

And all family members must take time to grieve. Some may benefit from talking to like-minded people who understand. Veterinary colleges have hotlines manned by students trained in grief counseling.

Help your child (and yourself) cope by encouraging them to talk about how much they miss their friend. Look at photographs of happy times with your dog and help your child plan a goodbye ceremony for their special friend. Well-meaning euphemisms like the dog "went to sleep" may worry some children about going to bed fearing they too may not wake up. Speak in clear yet simple terms.

Do pets grieve? You bet they do! Give your other best-friends time and grieve along with them. Increase your bond by spending quality time together. Just like us, working through grief takes time and every pet exhibits different behaviors. Some may sleep near the deceased pet's bed, toys or food dishes and appear sad while others may act as if nothing has changed. When the time is right, loving another canine family member can help heal the heart but never replaces the old friend you said goodbye to. Every dog will leave his own unique set of paw prints on your heart!

The Rainbow Bridge
Author Unknown but inspired by a Norse Legend

By the edge of a woods, at the foot of a hill,
Is a lush, green meadow where time stands still.
Where the friends of man and woman do run,
When their time on earth is over and done.
For here, between this world and the next,
Is a place where each beloved creature finds rest.
On this golden land, they wait and they play,
Till the Rainbow Bridge they cross over one day.
No more do they suffer, in pain or in sadness,
For here they are whole, their lives filled with gladness.
Their limbs are restored, their health renewed,
Their bodies have healed, with strength imbued.
They romp through the grass, without even a care,
Until one day they start, and sniff at the air.
All ears prick forward, eyes dart front and back,
Then all of a sudden, one breaks from the pack.
For just at that instant, their eyes have met;
Together again, both person and pet.
So they run to each other, these friends from long past,
The time of their parting is over at last.
The sadness they felt while they were apart,
Has turned into joy once more in each heart.
They embrace with a love that will last forever,
And then, side-by-side, they cross over… together.

Why You Should Know Canine First-Aid and CPR

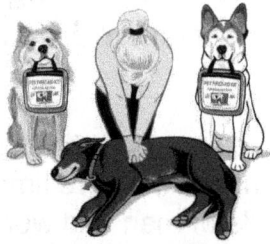

PET FIRST-AID & CPR
Saves Lives!

Image Courtesy of Sunny-dog Ink

Without warning, tragedy can strike, so you must know what to do when something happens. Have you ever driven down a dimly lit road to narrowly escape hitting an animal? Has an outdoor cookout ever tempted your pooch to reach up for a sizzling treat? Has a furry tail ever been accidentally closed in a door, or have you found ticks on your long-haired dog ? Did you discover a dog in a car suff ering from heat stroke this summer? How about vomiting, diarrhea and bee stings – have your pets ever experienced these problems?

Statistics show that preventable accidents are the leading cause of death among our pets, and 9 out of 10 dogs and cats can expect to have an emergency during their lifetime.

According to the American Animal Hospital Association (AAHA), one out of four additional animals could be saved if just one Pet First-Aid technique was applied prior to the animal receiving veterinary care. What this means is that the most competent Veterinarian cannot bring dog pet back to life, but by knowing Dog First-Aid & CPR, you can keep your dog alive until you reach professional medical help.

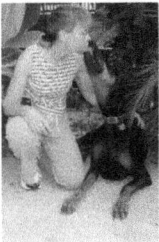

Photo by:
Shirley DeFazio

After a morning run along the beach in lovely Ventura, California, nine-year-old Rocco the Doberman collapsed on the driveway as he returned home with his owner Shirley DeFazio. Grateful she had taken a Pet First-Aid & CPR Class only three weeks prior, Shirley remained calm and got to work. Rocco wasn't breathing, so she checked his pulse. There was none, so Shirley began administering CPR. "Right away Rocco started breathing only to stop again, so I continued chest compressions and his heart started pumping and he started panting. He laid there calmly breathing until my little dog barked at something going by. Rocco got up all interested, ate his breakfast and stole my sock on the way up the stairs. I truly never thought I would use my training on my own dog. I can't believe I actually saved Rocco's life," Shirley exclaimed.

Although Veterinarians are the experts, they are generally not on the scene when something happens to your pet, so it is up to YOU to react quickly and eff ectively before professional medical care is available. Knowing what to do during those fi rst few moments can truly make a diff erence for your canine. What this means is that if you know how to stop bleeding and how to bandage a wound, you can prevent your dog from great blood loss and keep an infection at bay; if you can reduce your dog's body temperature, you can prevent brain damage and death, and if you can alleviate choking, you can stop your dog from going unconscious. Pet First-Aid is not a replacement for veterinary care. Together you and your Veterinarian should work as a team for the well-being of your dog.

Shirley was very lucky in that she actually resuscitated Rocco. In most cases of pulmonary and cardiac arrest (often due to heart disease, poisoning or severe trauma), we strive to keep the oxygen and blood flowing to our pet's organs until the Veterinarian can take over. If we delay, brain cells quickly die followed by the death of other tissues and organs. Therefore, knowing animal life-saving techniques and reacting immediately is a must for anyone who shares his life with a dog.

Pet Sitter Tina Kenny explains, "I was caring for two Cairn Terriers when one of them started choking. I am so grateful I had taken Denise Fleck's Pet First-Aid Class just the day before. I quickly took appropriate action and a biscuit shot out of the dog's mouth. There is nothing quite as rewarding as knowing I had saved the day for this helpless little dog, and her wagging tail and thankful licks let me know she felt the same way."

Baxter the Boston Terrier was having the time of his life, wildly chasing one of his siblings around his family's pool in Calabasas, California, when suddenly he slipped and fell in the deep end. Although the dog's family insists on yearly training exercises to remind all the dogs where the steps are and to be sure they can swim well enough to reach them, six-year-old Baxter apparently developed his own vertical style of swimming. "As Baxter kept sinking down, down, down, I jumped in to rescue him just as he was settling on the bottom of the pool," explains his harried owner. Her instincts kicked in and she pressed on Baxter's body forcing water from his lungs until he began to cough and breathe.

How It Differs From Human First-Aid

Instincts are great, if we listen to them, but very often since we're dealing with a species unlike our own, humans do the wrong thing or do nothing at all. Even if you have taken a human first-aid course, getting pet-specific training is essential since we do not share anatomies with our canine. The concept is the same in many instances, but the technique often differs. When giving rescue breathing to a person, we pinch off the nose and breathe into their mouth. It's the complete opposite for our dogs with us closing their mouth and breathing into their nostrils. How about compressing your pet's heart...did you realize that you must squeeze not only the rib cage but also compress the two balloons (aka the lungs) that surround the heart in order to effectively perform CPR? Since we can't ask our pets, "Where does it hurt?" or "What did you eat?", we need to constantly look for signs and symptoms of illness, and that requires us to tune in and really get to know our pets as well as learn the correct protocols.

Another big difference between human and canine patients is that animals might bite out of fear or pain. You must at all times be aware of your dog's changing body language so that an animal injury does not turn into a human first aid incident. You must know how to appropriately restrain and handle an injured animal and check the scene for any hazards before you begin tending to your precious dog because if you get injured, you will be unable to care for the injured animal. Furthermore, animals that are known to have bitten a person – even if the bite occurred during an emergency situation in which the animal was in pain – will require quarantine until rabies has been ruled out. Therefore, pet-specific training is essential for your dog's sake and yours as well.

Refer To Pet Safety Page 35 For Animal Body Language

By Knowing Dog First-Aid You Can:

- Lower your dog's body temperature if he suffers from heat stroke and prevent brain damage or death.

- Stop bleeding and prevent infection by properly bandaging a wound.

- Prevent your dog from losing consciousness by alleviating choking.

- Expel poison from your dog's system by properly inducing vomiting.

- Be the pump your dog's heart can't be until you can get him to professional medical help.

- By learning what can happen to your dog, you may prevent many emergencies from ever happening.

Nikki sat down in front of the TV for an evening snack and a scary movie with her Miniature Schnauzers at her feet waiting for a morsel -- their eyes wide open, ears pricked high with their hot doggie breath hitting her legs. She tossed them each a kernel of popcorn and the food-hound of the duo gulped it at the speed of lightning! Suddenly he opened his mouth, gagged and then stopped coughing altogether before going silent. Not only was the food lodged in his tiny windpipe, Nikki's furry child had stopped breathing! Fortunately for the Schnauzer, his owner knew how to perform the Canine Heimlich and the popcorn kernel flew out of his doggie mouth. Unfortunately though, he was quicker than his human and retrieved it, but this time swallowed without a problem.

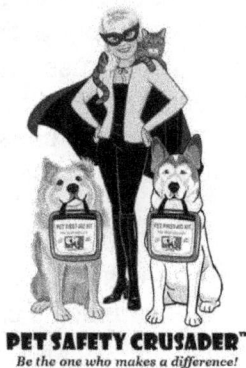

PET SAFETY CRUSADER™
Be the one who makes a difference!
Image Courtesy of Sunny-dog Ink

DOG FIRST-AID FOR INJURIES AND ILLNESSES

What is Dog First-Aid?

Dog First-Aid is the first thing YOU do to help a dog who is ill or has been injured. It is often the most critical step as it may dictate the eventual outcome. The goal is to make the animal more comfortable, lower the risk of infection and stop further injury before complete medical attention can be given.

In certain scenarios, after performing first-aid, you may just need to observe your dog until he heals, however, first-aid is considered the MOST critical step because in worse case situations, if your pet is not breathing or does not have a pulse, it could die before you get it in the car and to your Veterinarian's office. By knowing how to administer CPCR, YOU, can keep your dog alive until you reach your animal emergency center. If you don't jump to action at the time the emergency occurs, veterinary professionals may not be able to use their expertise to save your dog, for if they have expired…no medicine or surgery will bring them back.

Additionally, if you apply even one First-Aid technique, you may limit your dog's pain and time to heal and even save money. By controlling blood loss, you may avoid the need for transfusions. By limiting an injured pet's movements, you can prevent further damage to a limb which could result in a longer recuperative period and additional pain. These and many other reasons you will discover in this book (and in the course of being a pet lover) make it imperative that you learn Dog First-Aid. It is crucial for the health and safety of your dog and may allow him to live a longer life with you!

Finally, in every first-aid situation, be prepared to treat for "shock," so hone up on those skills on page 213.

Types of Emergency Situations: ABCs = Airway, Breathing, Circulation

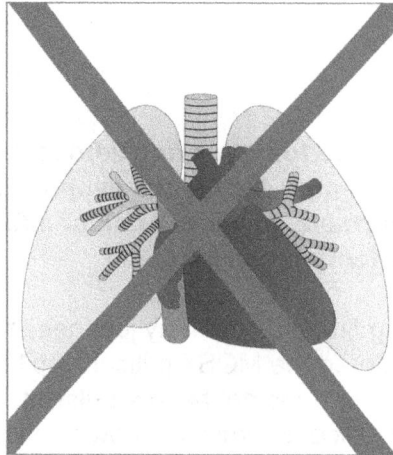

No matter if it's a dog, cat or human, these are the only three scenarios you will encounter:

1) **Heart & lungs are working but something is not right.**
   Distress may range from mild digestive upset to unconsciousness, choking, bleeding, seizures, etc. Depending upon the type of distress, this may or may not be a life-threatening situation.

   > You need to perform: **First-Aid** (the type of distress will determine the type of first–aid administered.)

2) **Lungs have stopped.** Heart is working (a pulse can be detected), but the lungs have stopped functioning. The absence of breathing should be considered a life-threatening emergency. Always check for breathing first. The rule is that if the animal is breathing, the heart is beating.

   > You need to perform: **Rescue Breathing**

3) **Heart and lungs have both stopped.** No pulse can be detected and the animal has stopped breathing. Within a matter of minutes, irreparable cell damage will occur. This is always considered a life-threatening emergency.

   > You must begin: **CPCR** -- Cardio Pulmonary Cerebral Resuscitation (Commonly referred to as CPR.)

Work as a Team With Your Veterinarian

How To Select Your Veterinarian

In addition to checking out your prospective Veterinarian's qualifications, make sure that he or she is someone that you feel you can talk freely with about your pet's condition and receive answers that are easily understood. Consider the expertise and experience with issues and conditions that your dog may experience. Take in to account your Veterinarian's inclination to consider a variety of treatment options and the Veterinarian's willingness to research and explain those in a manner that you can understand and feel comfortable with. Your Veterinarian should have a general concern for your dog's well-being and their office should not be so busy that it takes days to get an appointment.

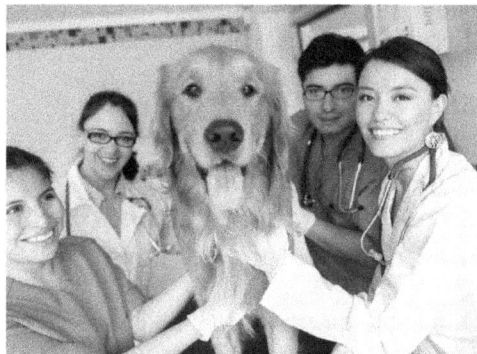

A Veterinarian should not only be competent regarding your dog's care, but they should also have a good bedside manner toward your four-legged family member. Ask around and listen to what other pet parents have to say. Check if your Veterinarian is a Fear Free® Certified, member of the American Animal Hospital Association (AAHA) and if the office is also AAHA Certified. Consider the obvious when visiting your pet's medical doctor. Is the office clean? Are there separate areas for dogs and cats? Is the front office staff helpful, attentive and friendly and do they remain at the facility year after year? Sometimes when the front office team changes frequently, it signals that something is not quite right at the business.

Remember that your Veterinarian is your dog's SECOND Best Friend (you, of course are number one) and plays a vital role as a key member in your pet's health team. Also see pages 9-12 for your Pet's Health & Safety Team.

Locate Your Nearest Animal Emergency Center

Some are open 24 hours; others open at 6pm and close at 8am the next morning to fill that gap of time when your Veterinarian is closed. Locate the one nearest your home, your favorite park or hiking location and wherever you and your pet spend time. Make sure you know exactly where the office is located, where to park and what entrance you will bring your pet in (if you have a 100 lbs. dog that can't walk, this can be of major importance). Know what services they offer (MRIs, transfusions, antivenin, ambulance transport) and how they accept payment. Research all this ahead of time because when an emergency happens, time can mean the difference between life and death for your pet.

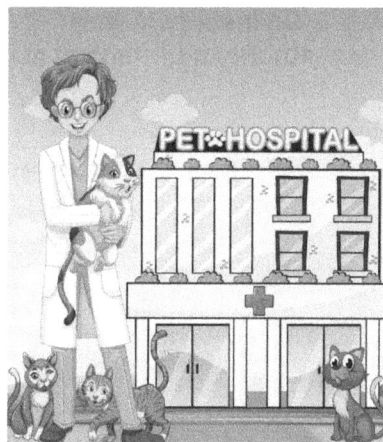

Needless worrying about which side of the street the Animal ER is on or what services they provide can be avoided by doing your homework. Being prepared applies to pet parents too and could save you time as well as your pet's life.

Fill in your important info in the back of this book on page 231 so that you have contact info at your fingertips when needed.

Most Common Situations That ALWAYS Require Veterinary Care

Regardless of what first-aid techniques you perform to alleviate pain and make your dog more comfortable, for the injuries below you MUST seek immediate veterinary care.

This list is by no means all-inclusive of situations requiring veterinary assistance, so if in doubt, always seek the advice of a licensed Veterinarian. Rather this list lets you know that if you have a dog experiencing any of these ailments, get him to your Veterinarian immediately! Details will be provided on pages to come as to how you can provide first-aid care to dogs for the situations listed below.

1) Anytime you have administered rescue breathing or CPR (even if he seems okay afterwards) or if the pet is having any difficulty breathing
2) Trauma to the head, chest or abdomen or anytime a canine has been unconscious
3) First-time seizure, seizure lasting more than five minutes, or in cases of an epileptic animal, a seizure lasting longer than is normal for that pet
4) Arterial or venous bleeding (major blood loss)
5) Fractures or suspected muscle/tendon strains or tears
6) Wounds more than 1" in length and/or more than ½" deep including bites and especially those which are prone to abscesses and infections
7) Suspected or known poisoning or snake bites
8) Shock (depletion of oxygen to the body due to blood loss, trauma, anaphylaxis or pulmonary/cardiac arrest -- a life-threatening condition you will learn more about in this book)
9) Inability to walk
10) Bloat (distended abdomen -- the animal can die within minutes)

For any of the above, do immediate first-aid and then...

GET TO YOUR Veterinarian AT ONCE!

Assessing Your Dog's Health

Learning to check your dog's vitals can help assess his degree of pain, injury or illness.

There are 5 vital checks that you should be able to perform.

The 5 Vital Checks:

1) **Pulse** – The rhythmic movement of blood through an artery.
   - Place the ball of two fingers (not your thumb) on the depression found in the animal's upper inner thigh over the femoral artery.
   - Count the beats for 60 seconds (or for 30 seconds and then multiply by 2 to determine his pulse rate.)
   - Take the pulse over 3-5 days to determine the baseline number for your pet.

If you have difficulty feeling the femoral artery, place the palm of your hand over the left side of his chest – just behind his elbow – to feel his heart beat which will be the same rate.

Average Heart Rate For Dogs	
Species	**Average Heart Rate**
Small Dogs	90 - 160 Beats Per Minute
Large Dogs	65 - 90 Beats Per Minute

2) Respiration – The process of inhaling and exhaling; breathing.

- Observe or place your hand over the animal's chest to count the number of times his chest rises (inhales) or falls (exhales). The "rise and fall cycle" should be counted as one breath.
- Count the breaths (rise and fall cycles) for 60 seconds (or for 30 seconds and then multiply by 2) to determine respirations per minute.
- Check respiration over 3-5 days on your pet to determine the baseline number.
- Do not attempt to count the respirations of a panting dog.

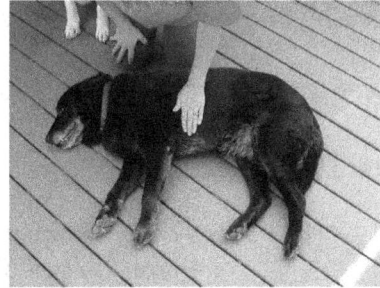

Photo by Sunny-dog Ink

Average Respiration Rate For Dogs	
Species	**Average Respiration Rate**
Small Dogs	**20 - 40 Breaths Per Minute**
Large Dogs	**10 - 30 Breaths Per Minute**

Please Note: *Very large dogs and geriatric animals may have slower respirations. Rule of thumb is that the bigger and older the dog, the slower his pulse or respiraton. The smaller and younger the animal, the faster their breathing and pulse rate.*

3) Temperature – The level of heat produced by the body.

- After lubricating the tip of a digital thermometer with petroleum jelly or other such safe product, lift dog's tail up to access the area and prevent him from sitting, and insert non-glass digital thermometer ½" – 1" into the rectum (slightly angled upward).
- At the sound of the beep or according to specific instrument instructions, the animal's temperature should range between 100.4º F – 102.5º F (38º C – 39.16º C). A temperature of 101ºF is considered average for dogs.
- A temperature of 103º F is considered a fever.
- A temperature of 104º F and above is considered an emergency.

NOTE: Feeling your dog's nose to determine his temperature or state of health is not an accurate measurement.

4) Capillary Refill Time (CRT) - The amount of time it takes for blood and oxygen to refill a capillary (smallest vessels transporting blood and oxygen throughout the body) after pressure has been applied and released.

CRT indicates whether blood circulation is sufficient to sustain life. Sometimes referred to as perfusion.

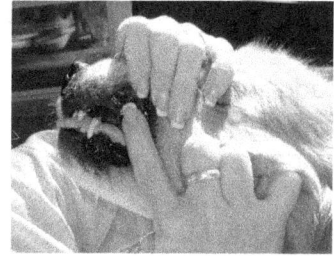

Photo by Sunny-dog Ink

- Gently lift dog's upper lip at the side of his mouth; it is often uncomfortable to pull up on the lip at the front and press on gums above teeth with the ball of your index finger until gums lighten. Be sure not to pull too tight because this can cause the gums to appear lighter and make it much more difficult to accurately assess CRT.
- It is best to choose a non-pigmented part of the animal's gums if at all possible, but if you only have dark gums to work with, you should still be able to determine CRT. If you feel unsure on a dark-gummed dog, gently pull down on an eyelid to see if the inside color is pink. If it is pale, seek immediate veterinary assistance.
- Release pressure and color should return to the gums within 1-2 seconds.
- If it takes color (blood flow) longer than 2 seconds to return to gums after you have released the pressure applied by your finger, increase circulation by slightly elevating animal's hind quarters with a pillow (unless there is significant bleeding to head or chest) and get immediate veterinary help. Also see shock on page 213.

5) Hydration – Sufficient water in an animal's body to sustain health. Dehydration is the loss of water and vital electrolytes such as sodium, chloride and potassium necessary for survival. The bodies of dogs are comprised of 70% to 80% water. As a reference, a 50 pound animal requires about 5 cups (or 40 ounces) of water daily, but if he's active that amount should be at least doubled. Dogs are resilient and can survive the loss of up to 50% of their muscle and fat, but a dehydration level of more than 10% is life threatening.

To determine adequate hydration levels, use the following procedure:
- Gently pinch a fold of skin at animal's nape of neck and release. The skin should quickly fall back into place if animal is well hydrated. This is often referred to as the Tugor Test.
- For loose-skinned breeds and older pets whose skin may have lost elasticity, carefully feel the gums. If they are dry or sticky, the pet may be dehydrated.
- Fatigue, constipation, increased heart rate and sunken eyes can also signal dehydration.

See page 240 for a chart to fill in with YOUR dog's vitals!

Head-to-Tail Examination

In addition to checking your dog's vital statistics, it is important to observe his body for signs of injury or illness. The more you know what is normal for any dog, the more quickly you will recognize something that is not.

Start at the head and work your way toward the tail, observing the skin and coat, feeling for lumps, bumps, abrasions and parasites. Notice any red or tender areas by also paying attention to your pet's facial expressions, movements and sounds. Dogs are more likely to remain stoic and tolerate a painful touch from a human.

Gently clean **ears** of dirt and waxy debris with appropriate ear wash and a soft cloth -- do not plunge a cotton swab into your dog ear canal as you could cause deafness or damage. Moisten a soft cloth or gauze square with dog-specific ear cleaner, ½ and ½ white or cider vinegar & purified water, or cooled green or chamomile tea to gently wipe out the ear. Do not use a cotton swab.... Also, do not pour the cleaner into the ear. First off, you may not get it all out as dogs have "L" shaped ear canals but additionally, you are flushing any debris in the canal down the ear causing it to then sit on the ear drum. If you discover redness, parasites or a foul odor coming from your pet's ears at any time, have your Veterinarian assess at once. What may look like coffee grounds could be dirt left behind by parasites such as fleas or mites.

New products appear on the market regularly, so check with your Veterinarian as to which ones are best to use on your pet. Remember however to always follow directions closely - dog products for dogs only, cat products for cats, and stick to the recommended doses according to body weight or other specifications. A small error could prove dangerous to your best friend. Also, watch him carefully when trying new products and observe his body's reaction to the treatment.

If eyes tear excessively or you notice a discharge, flush with eye wash (saline solution or purified water should be the only ingredient listed).

Compare one eye to the other for any differences making sure both pupils are the same size. Dogs have round pupils like we do and should respond to light by contracting and then dilating (or enlarging) when light source is removed. If pupils are not of equal size, your dog could have a condition and should be checked by a Veterinarian immediately.

Track your dog's eye movement by holding an index finger in front of his face and slowly moving it from side to side. Do his eyes follow your movements? If you detect any erratic flickers or jumps in the eyes, it could also indicate a neurological issue which a Veterinarian should assess.

Feel the **muzzle** for bumps and tenderness. Due to bone and cartilage, it may be impossible to feel a tumor, so if the area appears sore or if there is an unusual discharge from the nostrils, get to your Veterinarian for a thorough exam. Soreness on the muzzle, however, could also be coming from the mouth.

Do you brush your dog's teeth regularly? It only takes 48 hours for plaque to turn to tartar leading to gum disease. ***Carefully look in the mouth***. Gums should be a healthy pink (unless your pet has black gums like Chows and Black Labs) with no bad odor. Check for broken teeth and obvious signs of swelling or bleeding. Anything that doesn't appear normal should be evaluated by a Veterinarian. Sometimes small dogs are notorious for eating dental floss, string and tinsel which can wrap around teeth or the base of the tongue. Foreign objects that become stuck in the mouth should always be checked by your Veterinarian as they can cause inflammation or damage to the oral tissues. If your pet is suddenly losing weight or not eating, dental issues could be the cause. The rest of your head-to-tail examination should be a gentle massage along the animal's sides and back, looking and feeling for ANYTHING that does not belong -- abrasions, bumps, tenderness and sores; even parasites, burrs and foxtails that may have found their way onto your friend's furry coat. When you reach your pet's **chest**, you should be able to feel, but not see, the ribs. Breathing should be steady. It is important that you learn to check respiration and all of your animal's vital signs so you know you are doing your best for the health of your companion. See page 240 in this book.

Inspect legs and paws making sure claws and pads are not cracked, and keep nails trimmed so that they won't catch in carpet or break on concrete let alone scratch you or your pet. Be gentle and go a speed that is comfortable for your best friend. Many animals get uneasy when touched, but examine a little at a time, and they'll come to enjoy this bonding experience.

With your fingertips, stroke the **abdomen** making sure there are no hard spots or sensitive areas. Check nipples (males have these too), genitals and "under the tail" which should all be clean with no colored discharge. If your pet is older or arthritic and can't keep up with his own daily hygiene, help keep him clean with a warm wet cloth. If you notice scooting or excessive licking, the anal glands may need to be emptied by a professional.

Long or short, fluffy or hairless, the pet's tail should also be examined for bumps and sores remembering that the base of the tail often harbors parasites and that the tail does have nerve endings and a blood supply, so it can sustain injuries.

Throughout your assessment, check the dog's **skin and coat** for flaking or excessive shedding. The right brush can feel like a massage and help stimulate oil glands. If you notice anything that is irregular or abnormal for your pet, seek a professional veterinary opinion, and sometimes even a second opinion!

See Section III for Head-to-Tail Worksheet to keep you on track with home exams.

Also see page 232 in the pet safety section for a handy chart.

Basic Signs of Illness or Injury

During a head-to-tail check-up – or at any time – if you notice the following signs, the dog's health needs to be addressed. Don't be concerned about memorizing a list of symptoms. Think about when you yourself have not felt your best…what did you experience? It may not be that different from your dog except he isn't telling you that he is in discomfort. Canines are pack animals and it is in their best interest in the wild to not let on when they are hurt, so this often carries down to our domestic pets, especially if you have a multi-dog household. An animal who is injured or weakened can lose his place in the hierarchy, so he'll do his best to keep symptoms hidden. It therefore is your task to seek out anything that is not right with your dog through weekly head-to-tail exams.

In the pages that follow, you will learn how to deal with these situations. The information below is your check list for determining the basic signs of illness or injury in a dog:

- Redness
- Swelling
- Tenderness/Lameness
- Open sores
- Bleeding, pus or discharge from any orifice or wound
- Breathing difficulties
- Rapid or decreased heart rate
- Excessive panting
- Slow CRT
- Abnormal temperature or hydration level
- Frequent or infrequent urination
- Any kind of unproductive straining to urinate or defecate
- Vomiting/diarrhea/constipation
- Restlessness
- Inability to walk
- Distended abdomen
- Lethargy
- Change in eating habits
- Anything that is not normal for YOUR dog may not be right

Signs requiring Immediate Veterinary Care

Not All-inclusive but if you notice any of the following, seek immediate veterinary help:

- Severe bleeding or bleeding that doesn't stop in 5 minutes.
- Coughing up blood or bleeding from nose, eyes, ears, mouth or rectum
- Inability to urinate or defecate
- 1st time seizure or unusually long seizure
- Heatstroke
- Difficulty breathing
- Eye injuries
- Fractured bones
- Vomit / diarrhea with blood or recurrence (more than twice in 24 hours)
- Obvious pain or poisoning
- Staggering
- Refuse to drink for more than 24 hours

Remember that communication with your Veterinarian is always important and you should always feel comfortable seeking out their guidance, expertise and assistance.

Think Safety Before You Rush to the Rescue

You are no help to an injured dog if you get bitten or injured yourself. Take a breath and think. Kind of like you learned so many years ago, "Look both ways before you cross the street!" Prior to performing many dog first-aid techniques, it may be necessary to muzzle your pooch or wrap him in a towel in order for you to safely offer assistance. Even the sweetest of canines may nip when he is scared or in pain. Practice safety first and remember that animals are very perceptive, picking up on your emotions. If you do not feel confident enough to help, you are better off getting the dog quickly to someone who can.

Restraining & Muzzling Techniques

Rule number one is that you - the handler - must be in control. Make sure you have the dog in an enclosed area so that you are not struggling with him trying to get away while you are trying to treat an injury. In other words, make sure doors, windows, gates, etc. are closed and there is no chance for escape.

Dogs are predators and many will instinctually hide their injuries to retain their position in their "pack." Dogs tend to have a "den" mentality and may want to go hide to lick their wounds without the presence of a human or another animal.

Some small dogs settle best when you wrap them in a towel because it helps them feel more secure, but they may need to be muzzled to prevent them from biting you.

Generally the best form of restraint is the least amount needed. A commercially-made muzzle works best for Brachycephalic (flat faced) dog breeds. For others, a temporary muzzle may be made from a length of soft cloth or a roll of gauze.

<u>To Make A Temporary Muzzle:</u>

Photos by Sunny-dog Ink

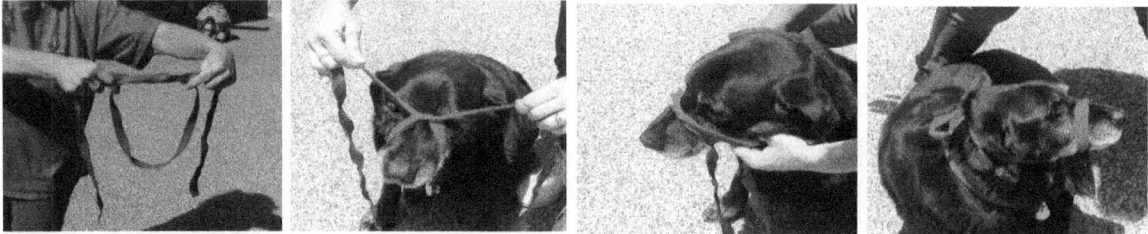

1) With a piece of soft cloth, such as a gauze roll or a strip of fabric, make a loop in the center of the fabric strip.
2) Slip loop over animal's snout and tighten to firmly shut mouth, but make sure fabric does not cut into dog's skin.
3) Cross ends of fabric under chin, exchanging ends in each hand.
4) Bring ends of fabric around each side of dog's neck and tie off in a bow – never a knot – behind the ears.
5) If the fabric strip you are using is long enough, it is best to do an added step. Just prior to tying your bow loops in Step 4, bring the longest end you have left across the crown of the dog's head and tuck the end under the loop made on the snout. Then bring the two ends back together and tie a bow (behind the neck is preferable but depending on your fabric, you may only reach the top of the head with the bow). What this additional step does is secure the muzzle in another location as well as pulling it tighter to the forehead.

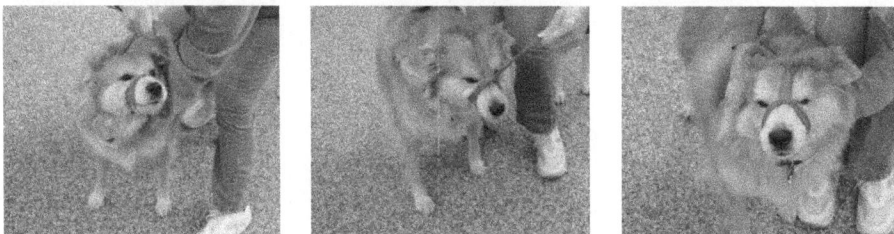

Photos by
Sunny-dog Ink

Never leave a muzzled dog unattended -- he is defenseless. If a muzzled animal experiences breathing difficulty, vomiting or seizures, they could easily suffocate. Remove muzzle immediately if such signs or symptoms occur.

Additional restraint can include tying a leash to a table or fence post so that you have control over the animal and use of both of your hands as well as just making sure the pet is securely leashed or harnessed. Any leash (if long enough) can become a Figure 8 Harness by looping once around the neck, and then bringing around the chest and securing by placing the handle through the "O" or "D" ring or the hook through the handle.

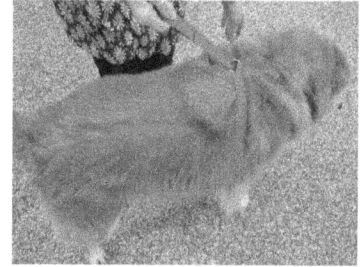

Photo by Sunny-dog Ink

How to Transport & Carry an Injured Dog

A towel or large triangular bandage can be placed under the abdomen in front of the hind legs as a sling to support a medium to large dog's hindquarters as you assist him walking. If the animal is immobile, you can improvise a make-shift stretcher by carefully sliding a towel or tarp underneath him. With the aid of another human, you can lift the pet by holding the ends taut to carry the animal to safety. If you happen to be alone with a large dog (too big for you to carry), use this method to drag the animal closer to help or transportation. Once again, slide the tarp or blanket gently under the pet, and on a smooth flat surface, pull one corner of the fabric carefully bringing the pet with it.

Boards of all kinds can be used as backboards if you suspect back or neck injuries. Plywood, an ironing board or a dolly can all be used to move a medium-sized dog. Carefully secure the pet to the board before lifting, tying him with torn sheet fabrics or rope, make sure towel or other fabric cushions him from ties or anything that could cause further injury.

For small dogs, if the animal is too injured to be placed inside a carrier, remove the top (if possible) or place the animal into a sturdy cardboard box with an open top. Although no one likes to think of their tiny pooch on a cookie sheet, small boards like cookie sheets, pull-out counter cutting boards and the lids from plastic storage boxes all make excellent boards to secure or small dog to. Just brace them at the hips and shoulders by tying with the triangular bandage or even gauze out of your dog's first-aid kit.

Do not attempt to carry a dog on any kind of improvised backboard device if the canine is struggling or resisting the restraint as this could cause additional injury.

Assembling a Dog First-Aid Kit

Just like a plumber or a carpenter, every task becomes easier if you have the right tool for the job, so aside from possessing life-saving skills, it is vital to have your dog's tool kit -- a Dog First-Aid Kit -- at your fingertips…at home, in the car, on hikes and in your disaster preparedness supply.

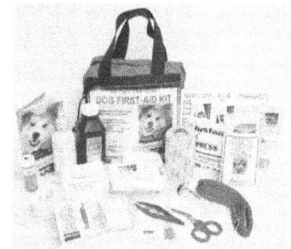

Photo by Sunny-dog Ink

All dog first-aid kits should include:

- 4" X 4" gauze squares to control bleeding
- Rolled gauze (varying sizes) to secure gauze squares in place, bandage a wound or make a temporary muzzle
- Adhesive tape or self-adhering bandage – to secure rolled gauze in place
- Styptic powder and cotton swabs to control minor bleeding
- Bandage scissors or blunt-nose scissors to carefully remove bandages, cut proper lengths of bandaging materials or safely trim pet fur
- Tweezers - to pull ticks or remove debris from a wound
- Hydrogen peroxide (3%) to induce vomiting or clean a wound site
- Eye wash or sterile saline solution to flush minor wounds and clean eyes
- Chlorhexidine (commonly found as Hibiclens®) to flush cuts and wounds
- Cold pack to aid in heat stroke, swollen joints, burns and bee stings (apply to site of injury but frequently remove to prevent over-chilling/frostbite to the area)
- Antibiotic ointment or Vitamin E gel or pure aloe vera gel to soothe and promote healing. Apply externally to minor cuts, scrapes and insect bites (not animal bites). If using medicated ointments, use the least amount necessary making sure it soaks in so that your pet does not ingest when licking because he will.
- Dose syringe (needle-less syringe) or eye dropper to administer medications and other liquids
- Digital thermometer to check your pet's temperature
- Antihistamine tablets (Diphenhydramine or Benadryl® - not containing cetirizine, acetaminophen or pseudoephedrine) for bee stings or allergic reactions (if you can find gel capsules, also have a straight pin in your kit to prick them open. You can then squeeze the liquid under your pet's tongue. Anything that is absorbed sublingually gets into the system even faster than swallowed.)
- Antacid tablets to soothe an upset stomach - Common pet emergencies are caused when dogs consume people food.
- Electrolyte solution to aid in re-hydration. K9 Quencher® and GoDog® are pet-specific products, but Pedialyte®-type products are fine as long as they do not contain xylitol, an artificial sweetener harmful to pets. Sports-type drinks contain too much sugar and are not recommended. Pedialyte® should be diluted with water 50/50. Having salt & honey to make your own is also a smart idea (see recipe on page 174).
- Nylon slip-leash to restrain a dog or devise a figure 8-harness. Can also be used as a temporary muzzle because even the gentlest of pooches may need to be restrained to safely allow care to an injury.
- Towel or blanket can be used to cover a pooch to maintain body heat and/or elevate his hindquarters to promote circulation. Can also be used as a temporary stretcher or a sling to aid a pet who cannot walk on his own.
- Honey or Karo® Syrup
- This Dog First-Aid Handbook to assist with the important details you need to know.
- Important names and phone numbers including your Veterinarian, nearest veterinary emergency center, animal poison control, helpful neighbors, police and fire departments.

HOW TO GIVE YOUR DOG AN INJECTION OR SUB-Q FLUIDS

These techniques are best learned from your Veterinarian, but as a reminder once you've been properly instructed...

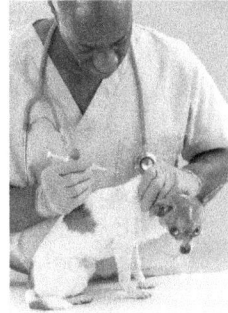

1) Draw the precise dose of medication into the syringe by placing the hub of proper sized needle into the vial's rubber stopper. Vial should be held upside down to a 45° angle for best effect.

2) Point the needle towards the ceiling and tap the syringe with your finger making sure any and all bubbles move to the top of syringe near the needle.

3) Slightly press the plunger on the syringe to force out any air. When you notice a teeny tiny drop of medication come out the tip of the needle, the air is out and you are set to inject.

4) Get yourself and your dog in a comfortable position and project calmness. Animals are very perceptive and will pick up on any stress you have. Gently pull up on the loose skin at the nape of your dog's neck or shoulders with one hand, while inserting the needle horizontally with the other. Take care to note your finger location and be careful to not insert the needle all the way through the pet's skin and into your own finger.

5) Smoothly press on plunger and release full complement of medication under your dog's skin, then remove needle.

6) Depending on the medication, your Veterinarian might advise you to rub the area afterwards to soothe the sting and help deliver the meds into your pet's body.

7) Properly dispose of needle in a "Sharps" container and give your dog a little extra TLC for being such a good patient!

ALWAYS use the proper gauge (size) needle and amount of medication as dosed by your Veterinarian and report any usual reactions to him immediately. FYI...the smaller the number, the thicker the needle!

For sub-cutaneous fluid injections, which are usually due to severe dehydration or chronic kidney disease, the technique is very similar to giving an injection of insulin or other medication, but is done in larger quantities. Due to the amount given, it may take several hours for the fluid to be absorbed, so always check at the injection site and at the belly to make sure fluids have been fully absorbed before giving another dose. The reason you also need to check at the belly is gravity which can cause the fluid to accumulate at the under carriage.

Again, this technique is best learned from your veterinary professional and may vary slightly from dog to dog, but as a reminder:

1) Place hub proper needle with plastic cover still in place over the tip of the syringe. Some brands have threads and actually screw together.

2) Fluids generally come in plastic bags or glass bottles. You may be instructed to draw fluids from the same container several times and/or for several days. Never re-draw fluids from a container that you have used to inject fluids into your dog or cat or you will contaminate the fluid! Always use a sterile needle. Using an 18 gauge pink needle to draw fluids and a 20 gauge yellow needle to inject into your pet will minimize confusion, but go on the advice of your Veterinarian.

3) Clean the rubber stopper or port of the bag with chlorhexidine or betadine. Alcohol takes 30 minutes of contact to kill bacteria, so it's not the best choice.

4) Lay bag of fluid on a flat surface, remove plastic cover from needle and insert needle into rubber stopper horizontally so as not to puncture neck of fluid bag. Never use fluid if it appears cloudy through the bag.

5) Draw into syringe the appropriate amount of fluid. Remove needle from stopper, place plastic cover back over needle and remove needle from the barrel of the syringe to replace with sterile needle needed to give the injection.

6) When ready to inject, push plunger to release any air and gently grab fold of skin along dog's back or neck with your left hand if you are right handed (southpaws reverse). Inject needle into skin making sure blood does not appear. If it does, you have hit a blood vessel, so back out needle and try again.

7) Once needle is in place, release the fold of skin and push on plunger to inject fluid. It is often helpful to steady the barrel of the syringe with one hand while you press plunger with the other.

8) Safely dispose of needles, properly store any unused fluids and as always... give your four-legged patient a special belly rub or ear scratch for being a good patient.

How to use a Stethoscope

Find a quiet space for you and your pet, then...

1) Angle the binaurals (ear pieces) forward so as to be at the same angle as your ear canal.

2) Moisten the pet's hair with water or rubbing alcohol to reduce the sound of hair rustling against the heads.

3) Have pet sit or stand. Lying on their side may cause the heart to rub against the chest wall. Place the bell (larger round disc) on the left side of the dog where his elbow touches his chest if it were gently pulled back. For smaller dogs, you may want to try using the smaller disc, the diaphragm, by placing it over the sternum (center of the chest).

Average Heart & Respiration Rate For Dogs	
Species	*Average Heart & Respiration Rate*
Small Dogs	*90 - 160 Heart Beats Per Minute* *20 - 40 Breaths Per Minute*
Medium to Large Dogs	*65 - 90 Heart Beats Per Minute* *10 - 30 Breaths Per Minute*
Please Note: Very large dogs and geriatric animals may have slower respirations. Rule of thumb is that the bigger and older the dog, the slower his pulse or respiraton. The smaller and younger the animal, the faster their breathing and pulse rate.	

HEART BEAT If you do not hear anything, administer CPR and get to your Veterinarian or Animal ER immediately! Swishing or a vibration could indicate a murmur, so please have pet seen by a medical professional.

RESPIRATORY SOUNDS Anything other than rhythmic breaths requires diagnosis by your Veterinarian, including wheezing, gurgling or whistling sounds. Don't delay.

Don't Just Stand There! How to Handle a Choking Pet

It was a picture-perfect Thanksgiving in Thomasville, Pennsylvania. A patchwork of red, orange and gold leaves blanketed the ground while a smattering of green still clung to the branches above. The house was filled with idle chatter while all anxiously awaited the holiday meal. Suddenly Brutus, a 90 lbs. Rottweiler, entered the room with an unsteady gait. Unable to breathe and making a ghastly assortment of noises, the dog was in grave distress while the humans nearby froze in a panic. Fortunately for Brutus, Animal Communicator Terri Steuben was on the scene and could sense the true emergency at hand. She quickly hugged the large dog around his abdomen and gave a quick thrust. Nothing happened, so Terri tried again, and this time a chunk of dog food literally flew out of Brutus' mouth and across the floor. The grateful Rottie, whose breathing returned to normal, began licking Terri's face as if to say a great big canine "thank you," while Terri herself breathed an enormous sigh of relief.

If your dog is destructive with toys, gobbles his food like Brutus or consumes everything in sight, you must maintain supervision and pet-proof your home. Dog Grandma, Milly Urbanski of Shadow Hills, California attests that, "My human kids had to put a child-proof lock on the refrigerator to keep their yellow Labrador Retriever safe. I was dog-sitting one morning, and the minute my daughter and her husband left for work, the mischievous pooch ran to the fridge, grabbed the bottom corner and flung the door open hoping to enjoy a buffet."

CHOKING

CONDITION OVERVIEW:
When an object gets lodged in front of the trachea (windpipe) instead of passing down the esophagus, it can prevent air from getting to the pet's lungs and can cause them to go unconscious – a life-threatening condition. Dogs are more affected than cats since they play catch and run with balls and sticks as well as chew on toys, rawhides, bones and other items that can be easily swallowed.

Never pull string, yarn or ribbon of any sorts out of either end of your dog. It could have something sharp attached to it or it could be caught on a nodule or other body part. Get pet to veterinary care.

PREVENTIVE MEASURES INCLUDE:
Get down on all fours and look at your house and yard from your pet's perspective. Anything in paw's reach could end up inside him:

Common Household Items that can be swallowed:
- Push pins, staples, buttons, rubber bands, toothpicks
- Squeakers and/or stuffing from pet toys
- Tennis and ping pong balls, marbles and coins

Common Surgically Removed Items from dogs:
- Socks, underwear & pantyhose
- Sticks, bones, balls & chew toys
- Corn cobs
- Hair ties & ribbons

SIGNS & SYMPTOMS:
- Loud noise or cough as an animal exhales
- Rasping noise as he inhales
- Gagging or retching as if trying to vomit
- Pawing at the mouth
- Drooling
- Outward stretching of the neck
- Staggering and eventually rapid/shallow breathing
- Pale/blue gums
- Collapse

NOTE: If the animal's tongue is swollen it may have resulted in choking due to a blocked airway; but the choking may have also been induced by an allergic reaction.

WHAT YOU MAY NEED:
You must remain calm and act quickly.

Possibly tweezers, forceps or in the case of large bones or a tennis ball, needle-nosed pliers to help remove object from throat. Be aware however that your doggie or kitty Heimlich-like skills most often help you come to the rescue!

WHAT TO DO:
Initially, give the dog a few moments to cough. The pet may expel the object on his own. If the cause of choking is not alleviated by the dog's own coughing action, a careful sweep of the mouth with your fingers to dislodge the object is recommended if the dog will let you safely do so. Make sure you can see inside the animal's mouth before you attempt to move anything. Do not reach without looking as you could push the object deeper, tear laryngeal tissue by pulling an embedded object or even get bitten.

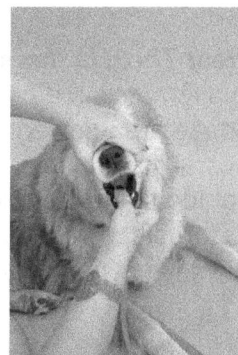

Photo by Sunny-dog Ink

Take care but, with hand over snout on dogs, cover their canine teeth by using your thumb and index finger to wrap their flews (lips) over the canines. Then use the thumb of the other hand to hold down tongue and lower jaw.

If the obstruction can't be safely removed, try one of the techniques below:

Lower Head to Expel Object

Place a small cat or dog on his stomach in your lap and lower his head in front of your knees. With the palm of your hand, deliver a firm blow between the shoulder blades to expel the object. Take great care with this techniques as spinal injuries could occur. Never use this method on Dachshunds, Basset Hounds or any other dog that is susceptible to back injury.

For a larger conscious dog, you can pick up his hind legs in a wheel-barrow method to attempt expelling the object. Do not try this if the animal is extremely resistant or showing visible signs of aggression. It is not safe to muzzle a choking animal.

Abdominal Compression, aka the Doggy Heimlich-like Manuever (for medium to large sized dogs)

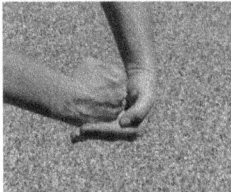

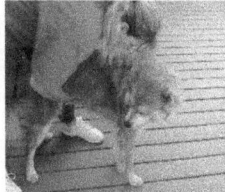

Photos by: Sunny-dog Ink

Stand behind your dog and place your arms around his waist keeping his head down. Close your hand making a fist and place your fist in the soft part of the stomach just behind the last rib. You should be able to feel a triangular area on his abdomen that would be the rib cage. Your fist goes in the center soft part of the triangle. Cover your fist with your other hand and compress the abdomen with 5 quick thrusts similar to the Heimlich Technique performed on humans. They key however to making this technique effective is that you must pull up against your own chest, so make sure there is no gap between you and the dog. His back must be right against your chest.

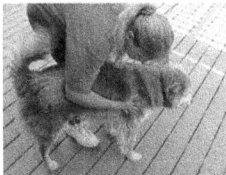

Photo by: Sunny-dog Ink

You may also try the Heimlich-like Manuever for small dogs using just the flats of two fingers (instead of your fist) in the soft part of the belly and bracing the pet with your other hand on his back, pulling up towards that hand.

Chest Thrusts (for small dogs)

An alternative method, especially for small animals since your fist may cover too much surface area (lower abdomen) in the Heimlich-like manuever, is to place your hands or several fingers on each side of the animal's chest and thrust inward, pushing with your shoulders and elbows in the direction you want the object to go – out the mouth. After 2-3 thrusts, give the animal a moment to cough and/or look in his mouth to see if the object is now reachable. If not, repeat.

Unconscious Choking Victim

Place dog on his side and thrust with hand over hand on just one side of chest to squeeze the lungs. By squeezing air out of the lungs, the goal is to create a force that will move the object into the mouth so that you can then reach it. Alternate these thrusts with rescue breathing & CPR if it takes more than 2 minutes to accomplish (brain cells start to die wihtin 3 minutes without oxygen) so get immediate veterinary help. Details are described in the next section for rescue breathing and CPR.

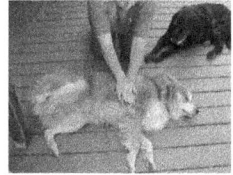

Photo by: Sunny-dog Ink

RESCUE BREATHING & CPCR

"I was driving along the bluffs of Palos Verdes admiring the houses wishing I could one day own, when I saw a dog hanging from a balcony! I ran up to the house frantically banging on the door and ran with the owner through the house. We pulled the dog up over the railing with as much caution as we could, and I checked to see that she was not breathing and did not have a pulse. Thanks to taking a Pet First-Aid Class with the author of this book, I knew what to do and started CPR. The owner left to call the Veterinarian and after about five minutes, the dog's heart started beating but still no breathing. Vet techs arrived at the house and hooked up oxygen whisking her off to the Veterinarian. After a couple days in intensive care, the dog came home and amazingly…is doing okay", explains Kim Kohler, relieved that she had learned what to do before she needed to know it.

	COMPRESSION: BREATH RATIO	NORMAL PULSE
NEONATES (Newborns)	1:1 Compress Chest 1/2" - 1"	120 - 200 bpm
SMALL (Under 20 lbs.)	30:2 Compress Chest 1/2" - 1"	120 - 200 bpm
MEDIUM (20 -50 lbs.)	30:2 Compress Chest 1" - 3"	90 - 160 bpm
LARGE (Over 50 lbs.)	30:2 Compress Chest 1" - 3"	65 - 90 bpm

CONDITION OVERVIEW:

Cardio Pulmonary Resuscitation (CPR) is the most commonly known method of artificial life support. Recent research has led to the advancement of a faster more efficient method referred to as **Cardio Pulmonary Cerebral Resuscitation (CPCR)**. Both of these techniques utilize a combination of chest compressions and artificial respirations, however CPCR focuses more on chest compressions and less on artificial respirations. CPCR utilizes the theory that the action of compressing the chest facilitates the movement of oxygen (that is already in the dog's body) through the lungs, lessening the number of times you will need to give breaths via the nasal passage. Oxygen moves through the body via the blood, so if you are promoting circulation, you are also moving oxygen via the bloodstream throughout the unconscious canine's body. Classic CPR uses a combination of five to fifteen compressions (depending on the size of the animal) and the administration of two breaths, whereas the more efficient CPCR procedure calls for 30 vigorous chest compressions for every 2 breaths given.

PREVENTIVE MEASURES/CAUSES INCLUDE:

- Smoke Inhalation
- Heat Stroke or hyperthermia (internal body temperature of 104° F or higher)
- Electrocution
- Hit by Car
- Drowning
- Poisoning
- Choking
- Gunshot
- Hypoglycemia (low blood sugar)

SIGNS & SYMPTOMS:

Dog has lost consciousness and both heartbeat and breathing have stopped.

Know that even under the best circumstances (in an animal ER with trained and experienced staff, medications, access to oxygen, tracheal tubes and IV catheters) the outcome may not always be successful, but how can you not try if a dog is depending on you? According to the American Heart Association, human survival rates range from 6.4% - 20%. In a hospital setting, on average 4% of dogs and and10% cats are successfully resuscitated via CPCR.

Although you may have taken a human CPR course, dogs don't share our anatomy. The concept is the same, but the technique is different. You may be familiar with the "ABC's of CPR" (airway, breathing, circulation); recent studies by the American Heart Association have shown that keeping the blood flowing to the brain (circulation) is more valuable as a life-saving tool than the administration of artificial respiration. In light of this research, the newest recommended protocol is "CAB" (circulation, airway, breathing) placing the emphasis on compressions over breaths . Following this recommendation from the American Heart Association, the veterinary community has also adopted this new protocol.

CAB = CIRCULATION, AIRWAY, BREATHING

WHAT YOU MAY NEED:

A hard surface on which to perform chest compressions (ground, table, floor, board underneath dog in a back seat for instance).

Calm, cool, you and the means to lift and transport the dog to the Animal ER.

Another person if available and willing to assist. Helping hands can be useful even if they are not trained in first aid or don't possess animal experience. As long as the person is calm, he or she can assist you in getting materials, lifting a pooch or even driving to the Animal ER while you tend to your dog!

WHAT TO DO:

- Place dog on a flat surface on his side and slightly extend his head by pulling back on the chin to stretch out his throat/tracheal area. Not only does this straighten out the airway but also minimizes your chance of blowing air into his stomach rather than lungs.

- *Hand Positions for compressions...*

  Latest findings by the American College of Veterinary Emergency & Critical Care, Cornell University, College of Veterinary Medicine, suggest using the *CARDIAC PUMP METHOD* for keel-chested (sighthounds) and small dogs by bending elbow back gently until it touches the chest to find location of heart. During compression on this area, the left & right ventricles are directly compressed delivering blood to the lungs and tissues of the body. During elastic recoil (rebound of the organs after compression), blood is drawn back into the ventricles.

  If the small dog is obese however, THORACIC PUMP METHOD may prove more effective.

- *The THORACIC PUMP METHOD* is recommended for square chested dogs and obese small canines. Place hands over widest part of chest to push blood from Aorta out to tissues of the body. During elastic recoil of the chest (as you stop compressing), blood is drawn back into the heart & lungs. This way, you are maximally compressing chest rather than just heart.

  For larger dogs, place the heel of the hand in the determined location (your dominate hand on top, interlocking fingers) and lock elbows keeping arms stiff. As you use your core muscles, maintain optimal compression force and begin your 30 compressions, rocking with your body weight up and over dog. NOTE: Not only are compressions less effective with bent arms, but by continuously flexing your biceps, your endurance will more quickly wane.

  For smaller dogs, it may be easier to feel at chest for heartbeat, then use two fingers to compress or sandwich your hand around (Taco method) to compress chest. See description on page 116.

- Compress approximately 1/3 the width of the chest diameter. You should feel ribs, then press a lung before you compress the heart to effectively create circulation.

- When giving breaths, use 1-2 hands to seal off mouth and breathe directly into the dog or cat's nostrils. For neonates, use a small puff breath only.

Never perform CPCR or rescue breathing on a conscious Canine!

CPCR Technique

For all medium to large sized dogs more than three months old:
1) Place dog on a solid surface with his right side down.
2) Begin chest compressions immediately, with 30 compressions at a peppy pace.
3) Follow the compressions with 2 breaths directly into the nostrils. You must make a tight seal with your mouth wrapping around the dog nose (see Rescue Breathing section which follows for details).
4) Repeat compressions.
5) The prevailing theory is "fast and hard" to do the job. Remember to compress 1/3 the width of the chest following the guidelines in the chart above.
6) Do not check the animal's status any sooner than 2 minutes unless there are visible signs of recovery.

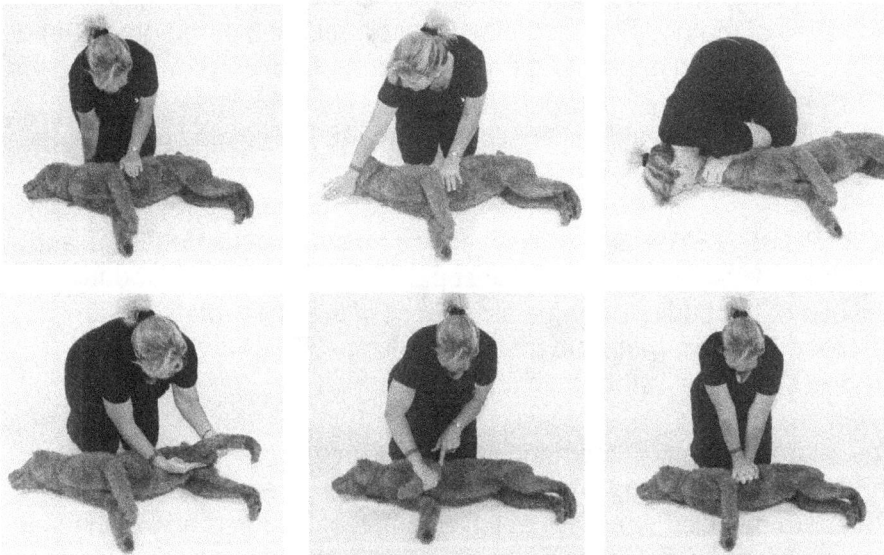

Photos by: Sunny-dog Ink

For small dogs and puppies less than three months old
Follow above CPCR technique but place their chest in the palm of your hand (use two hands if the animal's chest is too wide). Four fingers should be on one side, your thumb on the other side of the chest so that compressions will gently but directly impact the heart. Squeeze your fingers together to compress the chest. Follow with 2 breaths and repeat. Small dogs and puppies do not require as much

Photos by: Sunny-dog Ink

pressure during chest compressions but tune in and visualize to make sure you are applying just enough pressure to squeeze blood out of the heart then releasing to allow circulation and refilling of the heart before you squeeze again. You need to be the pump that the animal's heart cannot be at this time.

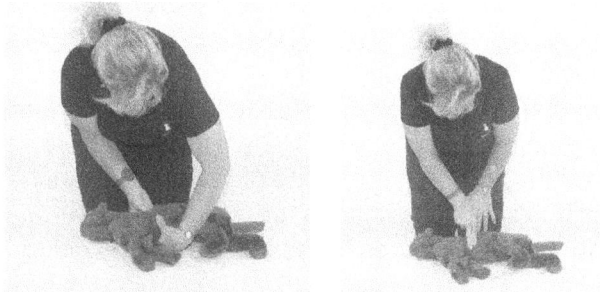

For neonates (newborn puppies and kittens -- hours or days old):
Follow the same CPCR technique as for small dogs, but administer one compression and one puff breath at a time. If your hand covers the entire torso (when trying to attempt chest compressions as mentioned above), place your thumb on one-side of the chest and use only two fingers (index finger and middle finger) on the other side. Squeeze the chest with the flat tips of your fingers.

Two-person Technique (works most efficiently in larger animals)
This technique is known as *Interposed Abdominal Compression* and utilizes one person performing chest compressions and providing breaths while the second compresses the abdomen cranially (towards the dog's head).

1) Person #1 administers 30 vigorous chest compressions as described above.

2) Person #1 administers 2 breaths into the nostrils at the end of each 30-chest compression cycle.

3) Person #2 compresses the abdomen on the "and" beats during the chest compression cycles (ie: "one-and-two-and-three-and-four-and," etc.). This pushes the blood from the dog's spleen and abdominal area towards the heart and brain.

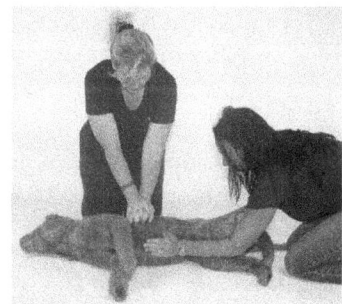

Photo by: Sunny-dog Ink

NOTE: Rapid initiation of CPCR is critical and must be started within 4 minutes after the heart stops beating to avoid brain damage.

Quickly transport dog to the nearest animal emergency center or veterinary hospital. Realize that you may not get the animal to breathe or resume a heart beat on his own and may need to continue CPCR while someone else drives. Do not stop administering CPCR until the pooch shows signs of recovery or until a veterinary professional can take over. It actually takes at least a full minute or more to perfuse the organs and tissues with blood and oxygen, so keep those compressions going to the best of your ability.

If you are able to continue CPCR on the way to the hospital, a firm floor like in an SUV or Station Wagon is best to lay the dog on. If you are doing compressions on a cushioned back seat, find a board or something sturdy to place between the pet and the cushion to aid squeezing the heart. Otherwise you'll just be pushing the injured animal into the seat cushion. If you cannot locate a board quickly, place your other hand/fist underneath the dog to press against. Remember...if you need to perform CPCR, the dog is theoretically "dead," so although we don't want to break a rib, the important thing is to get that life-giving blood & oxygen circulating. Properly performed, ribs break only 1.6% of the time which should give you some relief.

RESCUE BREATHING (aka Mouth-to-Snout Resuscitation)

CONDITION OVERVIEW:
Dog is not breathing. Lungs have filled with fluid, are in arrest, can't receive oxygen due to a blockage, swelling or other injury/illness. Dog is in a life-threatening situation!

PREVENTIVE MEASURES/CAUSES INCLUDE:
- Allergic Reactions (such as bee stings)
- Choking
- Collapsed or Punctured Lung
- Drowning
- Pneumonia
- Poisoning
- Smoke Inhalation
- Trauma

SIGNS & SYMPTOMS:
Dog is not breathing – no detected "rise & fall" to the chest.

WHAT YOU MAY NEED:
A calm demeanor (animals are perceptive and pick up on our emotions, even when unconscious).

Another person if available and willing to assist. Helping hands can be useful even if they are not trained in first aid or don't possess animal experience. As long as the person is calm,

124

he or she can assist you in getting materials, lifting the dog or even driving to the Animal hospital while you tend to your pet!

Means to lift and transport pet to Animal ER.

<u>WHAT TO DO</u>:
- Rescue breathing in our canine friends is done via the nasal passage (not the mouth as in humans). Their "smile line" goes farther around the face making it difficult to seal off the mouth and administer breaths without losing air through the sides of the mouth.
- Always make sure the mouth is adequately closed and sealed.
- Evaluate the size of the dog to judge the volume of artificial breaths to be administered. It is important that the lungs are not over-inflated. It is best to pay attention to your pooch ahead of time noticing how much his chest rises as he sleeps or rests to give you a frame of reference.

Rescue Breathing Technique

With the dog on his side, gently close his mouth with one or two of your hands until his "smile line" – the portion of his lips/flews that wrap around his face – are sealed.

- For a small dog, you may just be using your thumb and index finger to make this seal.

- Close your hands around the animal's nose and With his mouth closed, make a seal with your mouth around his nose so that you can blow directly into the nostrils.

Sealing a dog's mouth in preparation for Rescue Breathing

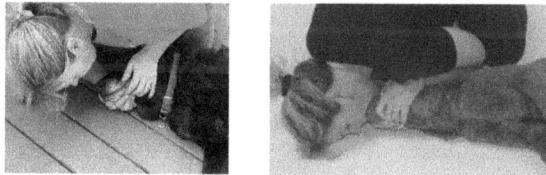

Photos by: Sunny-dog Ink

Deliver two slow full breaths into the nostrils, making sure you ventilate (actually see the lungs rise but just the slightest movement is sufficient) the dog and allow time for exhalation (lungs to fall into relaxed position) between the breaths.

Basic Dog First-Aid Techniques: Injuries & Illnesses

Now that you have a good understanding of vital signs, breathing, circulation and choking management, we will discuss the basic first-aid techniques for an assortment of other injuries and illnesses that could happen to an animal in your care.

Important…First-aid is not intended to replace professional veterinary care. The administration of first-aid is done in order to prevent further injury to the dog in your care and to alleviate pain and distress. Follow-up and continued treatment by a competent veterinary professional is imperative in most cases.

Familiarize yourself with this section for ease of use when you need it.

Like both the Choking & Rescue Breathing/CPCR portions of this book, each Injury or Illness has 5 sub-categories:

1) CONDITION OVERVIEW (explains the illness or injury).

2) PRECAUTIONS/CAUSES (how you may prevent and/or what might cause the specific injury or illness to help you assess if it is in fact what your dog may be experiencing).

3) SIGNS & SYMPTOMS (how your dog may be reacting if he does have this condition - he does not have to exhibit all the signs to be in distress).

4) WHAT YOU NEED (tools needed from your dog first-aid kit).

5) WHAT TO DO (action you should take, often including a trip to your Veterinarian) to help you help your pooch recover.

To assist in preventing the worst from happening, you will find more detailed precautions to take in the SAFETY Section in the front of this book. It is the authors' hopes that if you stay aware to what might cause injury and illness that you will be better prepared to help your dog avoid catastrophe.

A NOTE ABOUT HOMEOPATHY... Along with more traditional first-aid tips, homeopathic suggestions are offered in the Injuries & Illness section of this book. As with any other offering, your Veterinarian who has the luxury of physically seeing and knowing your pet is your best source for advice but listed are methods that may make your dog feel more comfortable prior to seeking veterinary care or with your professional's approval, along with other treatment.

Homeopathic remedies include tinctures, small pellets, pills and mists. Homeopathy works on the premise that "like cures like." For example, an approach to dealing with bee stings, rashes and other swellings would be administering *Apis Meliffica* which comes from the female honey bee (the females by the way are the only ones with venom). Homeopathy embraces the notion that the body can heal itself and that symptoms are a sign that the body is in a state of repair attempting to restore its own health. By giving a very small and diluted amount of a similar substance (herb, essence) the body's natural defenses are triggered to heal itself.

Homeopathics can often be administered along with other traditional treatments, and typically 30c of a homeopathic remedy is the highest dosage obtainable without a prescription. One "c" is equal to one part of the original diluted 99 times, so 30c is one part diluted 99 X 30.

Other identifying doses you may see include:

X = 1 : 9 dilution

C = 1 : 99 dilution

LM = 1 : 10,000 dilution

Best absorbed when placed under the tongue or on the gums, homeopathic remedies may be found as tinctures but also on sugar pills where just a drop of the remedy has been placed. It is preferable to avoid touching the pill by crushing it between two spoons and placing under your pet's tongue, or... to dissolve the pill in a drop of distilled water and then suck into a syringe to again be delivered under the tongue for best effects.

Once a good response is achieved with homeopathics, you do not continue with higher doses but back off frequency and amount.

Please Note:

If you feel uncomfortable performing any steps suggested in this book on a dogneeding care, instead...get the dog to immediate veterinary help. Animals are very perceptive and react to our body language and stress, so if you are fearful, it will be better for both you and the dog if you stay calm and obtain immediate assistance.

What you are reading in the following pages are suggested guidelines suitable for most dogs under normal circumstances. Your Veterinarian, Nutritionist, Behaviorist, Homeopathic or Alternative Medicine Specialist's recommendations should be taken over those presented in this book as that individual has the advantage of seeing your pet personally and knowing their unique history.

Injuries & Illnesses:

ABSCESSES

CONDITION OVERVIEW:
Abscesses develop when germs get caught beneath the skin as in the case of puncture wounds.

PREVENTIVE MEASURES/CAUSES:
- Animal bites/fights
- Nails, tacks, staples, splinters
- Gunshot

SIGNS & SYMPTOMS:
- Possible limp depending on location
- Hot, red, swollen area
- Open wound with pus
- Elevated Body Temperature

WHAT YOU MAY NEED:
- Thermometer
- Blunt nosed scissors
- Chlorhexidine, Betadine® or anti-bacterial soap
- Epsom Salt
- Gauze Squares
- Warm Water
- Warm Compress
- E-Collar to prevent licking

WHAT TO DO:
Carefully clip fur from area surrounding wound with blunt-nosed scissors, and wash away any discharge with a Chlorhexidine-type product. Soak a washcloth or gauze in Epsom Salt Solution (1/4 cup Epsom Salt to 1 quart very warm water), squeeze out slightly and place on top of the swollen tissue for 5 minutes three to five times a day. Wash as needed. Abscesses often become quite painful and need to be drained by a professional who can also prescribe antibiotics to heal completely, so see your Veterinarian. A blood test could also be necessary to determine if the infection has entered the blood stream.

NOTE: Never place a hot compress in the pits or groin area as you will overheat the animal -- these are locations to major arteries (Femoral/Brachial). If you can't avoid major arteries due to location of the abscess, seek professional medical help for your pet at once.

ALLERGIES

CONDITION OVERVIEW:
Pets can be allergic to many of the same things we are: dust mites, pollen, grasses and food. Often though instead of coughing or sneezing, dogs SCRATCH. They may also lick their paws or chew on their tails. An allergy is a hypersensitivity to something your pet comes in contact with. It is the way their immune system responds to what is irritating them.

PREVENTIVE MEASURES/CAUSES:
- Anything on the floor or ground can soak into your pet's paws or be consumed when he grooms. Using pet-friendly cleaners, insecticides and other products can help eliminate irritants.
- Avoid pet foods containing wheat, corn and soy as well as table scraps. Pollens, aerosol air fresheners and anything with a scent (remember dogs have much more attuned noses than humans).

SIGNS & SYMPTOMS:
- Scratching or licking
- Red irritated skin
- Hair loss in patches
- Sneezing, Coughing, Discharge from eyes or nose
- Change in skin or coat – flaky skin, dull fur; body odor

WHAT YOU MAY NEED:
- Oatmeal Shampoo
- Pure Aloe Vera Gel
- Diphenhydramine/Benedryl® (not containing Cetirizine, Acetaminophen or Pseudoephedrine)
- Possible change in diet
- Non-allergenic laundry detergent
- Scissors
- E-Collar or sock and bandaging material

WHAT TO DO:
A Veterinary visit and subsequent testing may be the only way to determine the root of the allergy and best course of action to take. If an irritation exists, you may try eliminating wheat and/or corn from your dog's diet (removing only one ingredient at a time for several weeks to determine which, if either, is responsible for the allergy), switch to a novel (unfamiliar) protein such as lamb or venison, and give Rover a soothing oatmeal or aloe bath.

Alleviate symptoms with Diphenhydramine (Benadryl®) – 1mg per pound of pet's body weight, but always check with your Veterinarian first to make sure it won't interact with any other conditions your pet has or medications he takes. Never use time-released capsules for pets. If using liquid Benedryl®, 5 ml should equal 12.5 mg of diphenydramine, so... dosage = .4ml / lbs. pet weight

For sore patches of skin, trim fur close to the skin with blunt-nosed scissors. Unless you are a groomer or Veterinarian, it may be difficult to use a razor on a moving canine without causing further harm. Clean the area with anti-bacterial soap, pat dry and apply aloe vera gel or hydrocortisone cream. Then prevent pet from licking or chewing, possibly by wearing the awfully named "cone of shame" (E- or cone collar. Do look around. There are many more comfortable versions available.). You might also try placing a human sock over the wound to prevent licking or apply a bandage with the overwrap containing a pet-safe anti-lick product.

ANAL GLANDS / ANAL SAC PROBLEMS

CONDITION OVERVIEW:
Has Rex been doing the butt-scoot boogie lately or has he been dashing around the house pausing only to lick his backside? Anal sacs are scent glands that normally release small amounts of fluid through tiny openings when your pet defecates. They contain a strong-smelling fluid that pets use to "mark" their territory and identify each other (Do you ever notice dogs checking their "p-mail" at the dog park?). From this information, they can tell each other's sex, interest in mating and what they had for lunch! When, for unknown reasons, they become impacted, infected or create an abscess, your pet scoots or licks to alleviate the discomfort.

PREVENTIVE MEASURES/CAUSES:
- Human food can cause stools to be unusually soft making fluid more likely to build up so avoid table scraps and make sure your dog consumes plenty of fiber.
- Doing a weekly head-to-tail check-up and paying attention to your dog's habits could alert you during the early stages before this condition, with unknown causes, becomes a bigger problem.
- Add 1/2 teaspoon for small pups or tablespoon daily of pumpkin puree or shredded raw carrot to your their diet. When the fiber is eliminated through bathroom habits, glands often express themselves.

SIGNS & SYMPTOMS:
- Chewing or licking obsessively under the tail
- Butt scooting
- Red or swollen anus

WHAT YOU MAY NEED:
- Rubber or Latex-free gloves
- Soft cloth or gauze square
- Shampoo or antibacterial soap for clean-up
- Pumpkin Puree or change of diet

WHAT TO DO:
Feed pumpkin puree (not pumpkin pie mix with added sugar and spices) -- 1 Tablespoon for a small dog and 1 Tablespoon for a large dog. Do not over feed the pumpkin as it is also a cure for constipation. Another option might be adding probiotics to your pet's diet. You should see improvements in about four weeks.

A temporary and much-needed fix however, is to express the glands.
Your Veterinarian or groomer should be adept at emptying these pesky sacs on your pet, but if you feel confident enough to try, follow these steps:

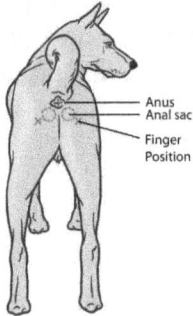

Anus
Anal sac
Finger Position

- Take your pet to the tub or a place that is easy to clean (Yep, this is a messy task).
- With rubber or latex gloves on your hands, kneel or stand at your pet's side, lift his tail with one hand and hold a cloth in the other hand to catch the secretions.
- For dogs…the sacs should be at about the five and seven o'clock positions around the main anal opening. If the sacs are full, you will feel two hard bulges, not much larger than a pea. With the hand that is holding the cloth, place your thumb and forefinger on either side of the anal opening at the positions mentioned above, and gently press inward and upward in a semi-circular motion as if tracing a clock dial.. Just make sure the anus is covered with the cloth. The fluid may be thin or thick and varies from yellow to light gray or brown.
- If nothing comes out, adjust your finger positions, but if you still come up dry, consult your Veterinarian. Pushing too hard may be painful to your pet.

ARTHRITIS

CONDITION OVERVIEW:

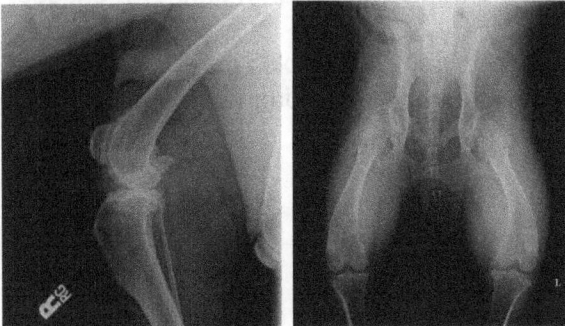

Degenerative joint disease or Osteoarthritis usually occurs after years of wear and tear on the joints but can affect a pet at any age. Large dogs are most vulnerable. It can affect one or more joints and is found in one out of five dogs at some point during their lifetime. Once your dog gets arthritis, he will definitely require veterinary care to alleviate pain.

Photos Courtesy of Sunny-dog Ink

PREVENTIVE MEASURES/CAUSES:
- Obesity
- Genetics
- Hip Dysplasia, Cruciate Ligament injuries, Patella Luxation can contribute

SIGNS & SYMPTOMS:
- Laying around more
- Pain or difficulty getting up; flopping when laying down
- Moaning with movement
- Labored, stiff movements

In some cases, constipation could be a symptom of arthritis! Since it may hurt your dog to get into the appropriate #2 squat position, he may not go and this may back his system up. The result is constipation but the cause could be the pain of arthritis.

WHAT YOU MAY NEED:
- Veterinary assessment to determine course of action (medication, therapy, light exercise, massage)
- Supportive pet bed (egg crate foam or firm mattress) in a draft free location. Too soft beds and nesting cushions are difficult to get up and out of.
- Non-slippery floor surfaces or toe/paw grips for traction.
- Back-end sling (such as the Gingerlead®) may assist walking

WHAT TO DO:
Keeping your dog at a healthy weight along with providing him regular gentle exercise to keep the joints fluid and the muscles strong is your best course of action. Slinging a towel under his hind quarters (behind his belly) or purchasing specialized slings and harnesses will allow you to assist your dog as he walks while taking pressure of sore hind joints

Make sure his dog bed is made of material he doesn't sink into too deeply making it difficult to get up and out of, and make sure it is placed in a draft-free location.

Raise feeding bowls so that larger dogs don't have to bend.

Provide ramps to make stair climbing easier. Placing a chair or low stool under a window will allow your smaller pooch to see outdoors. An ottoman or bench seat by your bed will allow your canine buddy to snuggle with you. So many new products are on the market to help out pets, so do your research and find what works best for your house and your pet.

Consult your Veterinarian for medications that may take the edge off his pain – for dogs, possibly a buffered aspirin (1/2 of a 325 mg tablet per 10 pounds of dog). Rimadyl, Carprofen, Deramaxx and Metacam work well for many pets but must not be mixed with aspirin or other meds. Follow your Veterinarian's instructions. New prescriptions often come to light, but always follow directions including any blood work or testing to catch any side effects early.

Glucosamine, Chondroitin, Methylsulfonylmethane (MSM) and Hyaluronic Acid are supplements that can help rebuild cartilage and joint fluids providing better movement for your dog. In 2018, researchers at Cornell University concluded a double-blind study on the effects of CBD oil on dogs suffering from osteoarthritis, an ailment not at all uncommon in our senior pets and people. Over the course of six weeks, dogs were given either CBD oil or an oral placebo, two times daily. Dogs who took the CBD oil showed clear improvement with veterinarians noting a decrease in pain and an increase in activity with no reported side effects.

CBD is an acronym for Cannabidiol (Can-a-bid-i-ol), a naturally occurring class of molecules called cannabinoids abundant in the plant genus Cannabis Sativa L. CBD makes up close to 40% of the plant and is just one of over 80 cannabinoids presently identified in cannabis sativa. CBD interacts with an animal's naturally occurring endocannabinoid system (more about this under "How does it work?"), and is non-psychoactive because there is little to no THC (tetrahydrocannabinol). In brief, CBD rich sativa plants having low levels of THC are referred to as Hemp and Marijuana plants are those with high levels of THC.

Speak with your dog's veterinarian about whether CBD could benefit your best friend.

BACK & DISC INJURIES

CONDITION OVERVIEW:

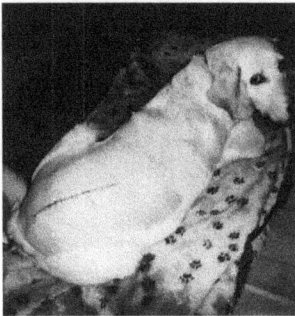

A dog's spine is made up of 30 vertebrae with 7 comprising the neck area. Back and disc injuries can occur from years of ill-fitting joints rubbing together or from traumas suffered.

Photo by: Sunny Dog Ink

PREVENTIVE MEASURES/CAUSES:
- Genetics (breeds with short legs and long bodies are more at risk)
- Overweight dogs more prone
- Provide ramps in place of stairs for Dachshunds, Basset Hounds and dogs with arthritis or joint injuries
- Falling, jumping, slipping or having an object fall on your pet
- Leaping on and off furniture

SIGNS & SYMPTOMS:
- Pain
- Inability to use hind legs or stand
- Walk with a wobbly gait or walk on the top of the paws instead of the pads due to loss of sensation

WHAT YOU MAY NEED:
- Pet Stretcher, flat dolly or... Improvise with a towel, board or surface you can carry dog on
- Triangular Bandage, strips of fabric or rope to secure dog to board
- Honey or Karo® Syrup
- Gauze and bandaging supplies

WHAT TO DO:

Get the pet veterinary help without causing further injury.

Check for breathing & pulse administering any first-aid or life-saving measures needed if injury was due to trauma (ie: stop bleeding, rub honey on the gums, treat for shock).

Slide flat board under the animal, keeping him as still as possible (Remember a calm soothing voice). Prevent movement as much as possible as struggling can damage the spinal cord. Secure the animal to the board with a triangular bandage or torn strips of cloth at the shoulders and hips. Place a towel over your pet's body and use fabric of rope over the towel to the board or other surface to keep him secure. The last thing you want is for your pet to fall from the stretcher as you carry him.

If dog is too heavy to lift, and you don't have a helping hand, you can pull the dog closer to the car by placing a blanket or tarp underneath him and gently pulling in the direction you need to go. You need to be sure that the surface you're pulling him across is smooth and free of sharp objects.

Transport to a veterinary facility immediately.

NOTE: A big part of first-aid is doing the best with what you have at your disposal...for a tiny dog, a cookie sheet or cutting board can serve as a back board; an ironing board, boogie board or flat dolly for a larger animal. You can even make a stretcher out of a tightly stretched towel or blanket held by two people. Please read section on how to transport an injured dog on page 111.

BALANCE (Loss of)

CONDITION OVERVIEW:
Known as Vestibular Syndrome, the symptoms can be upsetting to see when your precious pet is experiencing a loss of balance. It is often mistaken for poisoning, seizures or even a stroke and sometimes…there is never a definable cause. In medical speak, when Veterinarians can't determine the reason, the disease or syndrome is tagged idiopathic. Vestibular Syndrome can strike a pet at any age, but older ones are more prone.

What the Vestibular system does is helps the animal stay in equilibrium in relation to gravity. It conveys information to the muscles and controls eye movement so that images remain steady and in focus. This all takes place through mechanoreceptors found in the inner ear. Therefore, inner ear infections are a known cause for vestibular syndrome in dogs and must be ruled out by your Veterinarian. Less common is a tumor on or near the Vestibular center of the brain stem.

PREVENTIVE MEASURES/CAUSES:
- Check your dog's ears weekly for signs of infection or debris and keep them clean.

SIGNS & SYMPTOMS:
- Head tilt, circling or falling all directed toward the same side
- Jerking of the eyes from side-to-side (aka Nystagmus)
- Vomiting
- Loss of appetite

WHAT YOU MAY NEED:
- Antacid prescribed by Veterinarian or 1 tsp Mylanta® for every 10-15 lbs. dog weighs to curb nausea
- Needle-less syringe or eye dropper to administer antacid
- Due diligence to make sure your wobbly dog doesn't fall or roam stray; secure windows, add gates to block off stairs and balconies and assess your home from your dog's point of view.

WHAT TO DO:
Get an immediate and thorough veterinary exam.

If the ear is found to be infected, treatment will be prescribed.

If the ear is free of infection, then you and your Veterinarian will determine if an MRI or CT Scan is advisable to rule out a tumor, or if the symptoms should be dealt with as if idiopathic in origin. Often the syndrome resolves on its own over the course of several weeks, and unfortunately there is no way to speed recovery. Anti-nausea and/or dizziness medications may be prescribed as well as fluids, especially if your furry patient cannot eat.

During this time, you must keep your dog safe by making sure they can't fall down stairs, out open windows, off balconies or other such hazards, and never let your pet with vestibular syndrome roam freely outside.

BIRTHING PROBLEMS (Dystocia)

CONDITION OVERVIEW:
Although it is important to have your Vet help you through a lady dog's pregnancy, you probably won't need to hire a Lamaze Coach. Do remember though all those dogs out there that never find permanent loving homes, and please spay and neuter your pets! The vast majority of births go smoothly, so resist the urge to step in unless you are really needed.

PREVENTIVE MEASURES/CAUSES:
- A planned C-section is preferable to an emergency one, so if you have a breed that is at-risk, plan ahead. Nothing is worse for the mom-to-be than to have to be rushed to the vet hospital in the middle of the night or to become exhausted because she has been unsuccessfully straining to deliver puppies, sometimes for hours. The puppies are more likely to survive if they haven't been stuck in the birth canal or had their placentas detached, so talk with your Veterinarian about the possibilities ahead of time.
- The Bulldog and Pekingese are examples of breeds who often benefit from a C-section, but other brachycephalic breeds (dogs with flatter pushed-in faces) also have difficulty whelping naturally because of their pups' large head relative to their narrow pelvis. There are however, non-brachycephalic breeds that are prone to uterine inertia (when contractions are not forceful enough) or who lack sufficient pushing ability to deliver puppies, so a C-section is often safer for them and their newborns. They include but are not limited to: Border Terriers, Boston Terriers, Boxers, Brussels Griffons, Bulldogs, Bullmastiffs, Chihuahuas, Cocker Spaniels, Dachshunds, English Toy, Spaniels, French Bulldogs, Neapolitan Mastiffs, Pekingese, Pomeranians, Pugs, Scottish Terriers and Yorkshire Terriers.
- If your dog is not an at-risk breed, that doesn't mean she won't need surgery to deliver her pups safely. Litters consisting of just one puppy and litters containing an oversized puppy just might require a C-section and can be determined ahead of time through x-rays carefully obtained by your Veterinarian, so…remember to be a team player with your medical professional for the sake of your four-legged friend.

SIGNS & SYMPTOMS TO CALL THE VETERINARIAN RIGHT AWAY:
- Your dog passes a dark green fluid before delivery which means the puppy lifeline (the placenta) may have become separated too soon.
- Your dog has been straining hard without delivering for more than an hour – the baby could be too large or in the wrong position to come out without assistance.
- Typically breeds with large heads and narrow hips need to have a C-section performed by your Veterinarian.
- Your female seems weak, nervous or restless for more than a half hour after the labor stops. There could still be another puppy waiting to see the world.
- Momma has muscle tremors days or weeks after giving birth, begins to vomit or has trouble standing up. These could be a sign of Eclampsia – a dangerous deficiency of calcium that sometimes occurs after giving birth.

WHAT YOU MAY NEED:

- Thermometer
- K-Y® or other water soluble jelly
- Disposable gloves
- Clean towels, lots of them and small ones like washcloths
- Blunt scissors or electric clippings for trimming fur
- Sharp Scissors for umbilical cord
- Iodine
- Rubbing alcohol
- Thread
- Bulb suction syringe
- Milk replacer, nursing bottles, eye dropper or needle-less syringe

SIGNS & SYMPTOMS THAT DELIVERY IS IMMINENT:

- Mammary gland enlargement and milk secretion (1 to 2 weeks prior to delivery)
- Restlessness, seeking seclusion, losing weight, nesting (12 to 24 hours prior to delivery)
- Rectal temp decreases to less than 99°F (8 to 24 hours prior to delivery)
- Straining & involuntary contractions of the abdominal muscles (Final stage as fetuses begin to move through the birth canal)

WHAT TO DO & WHEN YOU SHOULD OFFER ASSISTANCE:

If delivery hasn't occurred by 67th day, get to your Veterinarian.

If the neonate comes out only part-way despite the mom's efforts, grasp the emerging puppy with a clean wash cloth and gently pull him free. Do not attempt to remove a neonate in this way if you cannot see both the front legs and head.

If mom doesn't instinctively tear off the amniotic sac within 30 seconds, carefully peel away the amniotic sac from around the neonate's face. Clean the mucus from puppy mouth with your finger and then rub newborn vigorously with a clean cloth.
Encourage mom to lick her baby and sever the umbilical cord.
Mom doesn't bite the umbilical cord within one minute. This typically happens when the mother doesn't immediately remove the amniotic sac. To sever the umbilical cord, tie two pieces of embroidery thread (dipped in rubbing alcohol) around the umbilical cord. The first thread should be tied about 1 ½ inches from the tummy and the second should be tied about an inch farther down the umbilical cord from the first thread. Clean a pair of sharp bandage scissors with rubbing alcohol and snip the umbilical cord between the threads.

HOMEOPATHIC TIP:

If the pet is having difficulty with discharges, such as after a false pregnancy or following pyometra, *Pulsatilla* may be useful. Consult your Homeopathic Veterinarian in advance.

BLADDER CONTROL PROBLEMS

CONDITION OVERVIEW:
Incontinence occurs when your dog cannot voluntarily control the act of voiding their urine. Bladder control problems can be related to infections and kidney disease, so a trip to your pet's medical professional is the best place to start. Incontinent pets wet their beds, the floor where they nap, dribble urine and go in inappropriate places even when they know better. This is often seen in older pets and can be caused by an estrogen (females) or testosterone (males) deficiency since these hormones play a role in the muscle tone of the urethral sphincter. Additionally, males with prostate issues don't completely empty their bladders when they answer nature's call, so they are always partially full and feel the urge to go more frequently, and sometimes...just can't reach the appropriate location in time.

Urinating in the wrong place however, can sometimes but a behavioral issue due to a change or disruption in lifestyle. Is a new pet now sharing the house, or has work been keeping you away longer hours? Does your dog become timid when you raise your voice or overly excited when you arrive home? All of these situations can cause certain pets to go right then and there or seek out your new bedspread to take out their frustrations on. Ask your Veterinarian to refer you to an Animal Behaviorist if you are seeing a pattern and medical conditions have been ruled out.

PREVENTIVE MEASURES/CAUSES:
- Diabetes or Hypothyroidism
- Weakened muscle tone due to hormonal changes or age
- Prostate issues
- Urinary Tract Disease
- Stones, crystals or debris accumulate in the bladder or urethra
- Tumors
- Spinal cord problems

SIGNS & SYMPTOMS:
- Damp or wet bedding or sleeping area
- Straining or crying when attempting to go
- Skin around genitals appears red/sore from the ammonia-like leaking; constant licking of the area
- Bloody or cloudy urine
- Increased thirst
- Increased frequency in visits to the litter box or asking to go outside

WHAT YOU MAY NEED:
- Veterinary visit for starters to diagnose problem.

WHAT TO DO:

Allow dogs more opportunities to go out and answer nature's call. A doggie door to a securely fenced yard may assist.

Take up water bowls two-hours before "lights out" and keep meals on a regular schedule.

Make any clean-up easier for you so that you won't become frustrated with your precious dog.

Line bedding with plastic and make sure everything is easily washable -- no dry clean only materials.

Doggie diapers can be worn but check them frequently so that irritating fluids don't scald your dog's skin.

BLEEDING INJURIES

CONDITION OVERVIEW:

Arteries are the largest blood vessels that carry oxygen-rich blood from the heart to various parts of the body. Veins are thinner vessels that carry blood back towards the heart while Capillaries are the smallest of all blood vessels. Capillaries are so small, that sometimes only a few red blood cells can pass through the center of the capillary at a time, so...if you have to see bleeding on your beloved pet, you should hope for Capillary Bleeding. They connect arteries to veins and near the surface can be found in the mucus membranes (gums, eyelids, ears and surface). Most of the time capillaries ooze rather than bleed, and mostly require superficial cleaning, antibiotic ointment and maybe a bandage to keep dirt and infection at bay.

From an artery, blood spurts as it is coming directly from the pump...the heart. It will be bright red in color since it is well-oxygenated coming from the lungs and there may be a lot of it! Controlling blood loss, bandaging to prevent infection and getting veterinary treatment all need to be accomplished quickly.

Since veins too are large vessels, much blood loss can occur. Generally, the blood is a little darker in color as it has given up oxygen on its return route to the lungs and has picked up toxins along the way. The blood will pool rather than spurt as it is not feeling the pressure of the heart pump, but same protocol is in order as for an artery...control bleeding, bandage to prevent infection and quick veterinary attention.

PREVENTIVE MEASURES/CAUSES:

- Get down on all fours in your house and yard and watch for sharp items that could cut a paw, catch on an ear or tail or poke an eye.
- Keep nails well-trimmed as a long nail can break and cause severe bleeding.
- Obedience and leash train pets, keep dogs in a securely fenced yard to avoid fights (and therefore puncture wounds) with other dogs and to prevent dogs from being hit by cars. Make sure ears, tails and other body parts don't get squeezed in doors (house or car).

SIGNS & SYMPTOMS:
- Appearance of blood whether it's oozing, pooling or spurting.
- If blood appears under the skin like a pocket or sack, this is called a Hematoma and requires a veterinary aspiration of the blood. If delayed, surgery may be required. Most commonly occurs in floppy ears that are scratched or bang a wall or table when a dog shakes his head.

WHAT YOU MAY NEED:
- 4 X 4 Gauze Squares
- Gauze Roll
- Blunt-Nosed Scissors to cut bandage materials as well as trim fur around wound
- Purified Water, Eye Wash (saline), Antibacterial soap, Chlorhexidine
- Antibacterial cream or gel (Neosporin®-like product) or pure aloe vera gel
- Towels, phone book or pillow to elevate injured areas higher than the dog's heart
- Miscellaneous old socks, pieces of panty hose, t-shirts, children's garments to help secure bandage around head, chest or tail

WHAT TO DO:
For minor cuts and scrapes:

Trim fur with blunt-nosed scissors to reveal wound.

Flush with water, saline solution, eye wash, antibacterial soap or Chlorhexidine (Hibiclens®)

Pat dry and apply antibacterial ointment or pure aloe vera gel to promote healing. Apply just enough to cover wound so that it will soak in, not leaving excess to be licked off.

If the dog starts to lick wound, bandage (see pages 142 - 144) or apply a cone collar to prevent pet from getting to injury. Using the self-adhering wrap that contains an anti-lick taste often helps. Try it yourself, it's icky LOL

For bleeding toe nails, pour dime to quarter-sized amount of styptic powder into the palm of your hand and press bleeding toe nail into the powder, also applying direct pressure against your palm until the bleeding stops. Watch for any signs of infection (redness, swelling, oozing or heat).

For severe bleeding injuries to the legs or limbs there are 3 courses of action to be taken to stop bleeding and promote clotting:

1) Apply direct pressure with gauze squares directly over the wound. If that alone doesn't stop the bleeding…

2) Elevate the limb by placing a pillow or folded towel underneath the injured body part keeping it higher than the dog's heart. If you still need help getting the bleeding to stop…

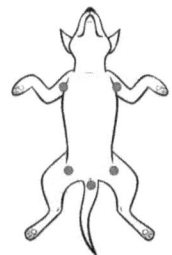

Image Courtesy of
Sunny-dog Ink

3) Apply pressure to one of 5 pressure points on your dog .
   Pressure points are arteries located closest to the surface of
   the skin, so applying pressure on the one corresponding to the
   injury, will lessen blood loss. (Think of a straw…if it's fully open,
   you can get the good stuff through, but if you squeeze it flatter, less will flow.
   The same applies to blood and oxygen travelling through your pet's blood
   vessels.)

FRONT LEG (Brachial Artery) – Place your thumb on the outside of the upper leg and your fingers on the inside close to the armpit to reduce blood flow and allow clotting to occur.

HIND LEG (Femoral Artery) – Turn pup on his back or side if possible, place two fingers at the stifle or knee and slide your fingers into the upper fleshy thigh near where his leg meets his groin. Press.

TAIL (Caudal Artery) – Steady a medium or large dog by kneeling and holding him against you (head towards your rear) with one arm over his back and around his belly. With your other hand, lift the tail and apply pressure firmly with your thumb on top of the tail (at the base where it meets the body) and two or three fingers underneath the tail.

For small dogs, hold them firmly in your lap against your chest while doing same technique.

Once bleeding stops, wrap flat gauze with rolled gauze, overlapping each layer by about ¾ widths each time around the leg, then secure with self-adhering elastic bandage making sure you can slip a finger underneath so as not to cut off circulation, then get professional medical help.

NOTE: Be patient. Realize bleeding could take 5 - 10 minutes, however if excessive blood loss is occurring, do your best to keep direct pressure and quickly transport the canine patient to the nearest veterinary office. If the bandage is too tight, it's unlikely you'll see skin turning blue, as in humans. With dogs, you are more likely to notice swelling above or below the bandage if it is too tight, or coolness to the skin below the bandage (as it is not receiving sufficient blood flow). Stay alert and loosen if you observe either.

BANDAGING TIP: After gauze is securely covered, just once take the gauze roll around the lower abdomen (when bandaging a hind leg) or once around the chest for the front leg, and then back around wound area. This creates "suspenders" -- a method to hold the bandage up. Legs are like vertical poles, and if the bandage is only wrapped around the leg, it can slide down once the dog stands.

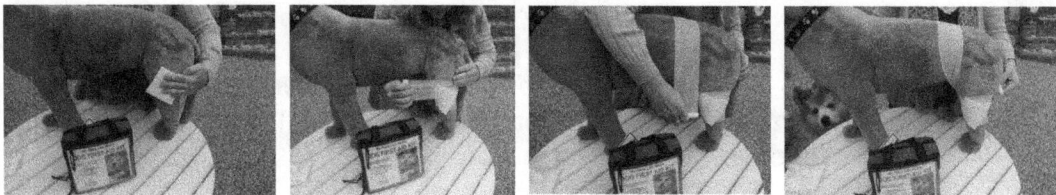

Photos by: Sunny-dog Ink

Never apply a tourniquet to control severe bleeding unless it's the only way to save a life, knowing that the paw or leg below the tourniquet will probably require amputation.

NOTE: In a situation where bleeding is profuse, if all you have is a clean towel, apply that to the wound and with someone else driving, continue to hold the towel and get the dog as quickly as possible to the Veterinarian. It's always wise to call ahead so that Veterinarian technicians can be ready to assist you.

Paw Pad Wounds
- Remove obvious debris and flush to clean if it's oozing, but if bleeding profusely, stop blood loss.
- Elevate to aid direct pressure and/or apply pressure to appropriate pressure point.
- Wrap paw with gauze encircling pad, and then between each of the toes - in a figure eight pattern - to hold it in place.
- Secure firmly but not tight with self-adhering wrap. This is especially helpful if a larger dog now has to walk to the car on the injured paw. The self-adhering wrap has texture and will provide traction.
- An alternative would be to slip a human sock over the bandage to keep it in place.

After treatment at your Veterinarian's office, you will be told to keep bandaging dry. When your dog goes out to answer nature's call, you may wrap a plastic baggie (the newer press and seal food storage products often do the trick) over the bandage and secure it with a little self-adhering wrap, making sure some of that wrap goes under the paw pad to give him traction on wet grass or slippery surfaces. It is imperative however, that when he comes in, you must remove the baggie. Dogs release heat through the pads of their feet, and need a bandage that breathes. Don't let bacteria breed in the bandage by leaving the plastic on.

Tail Injuries
- Apply direct pressure with gauze pad to tail wound, and lift tail to elevate.
- If needed, press on pressure point (Caudal Artery) at base of tail (where tail meets body) to diminish blood flow.
- Wrap tail with gauze roll to secure flat pad, then slip a child's-size cotton tube sock or leotard leg over the gauze roll.
- To further secure, if you deem necessary, beginning at tip of tail, wrap sock in a criss-cross pattern with adhesive tape going up the tail and 2" beyond sock and directly onto fur.
- Complete by criss-crossing back down the tail being careful not to wrap too tightly.

Ear Injuries

- For direct pressure...Think Opposites! Apply gauze square to bleeding and then press "upright" ears down towards the side of the face or check. For floppy "downward" ears, flip them up (wherever they fall naturally) onto the neck or top of the head for direct pressure.
- Ears are higher than heart so you have built-in elevation!
- No pressure on arteries as we don't want to cut off blood to the brain.
- Bandage in place using the good ear as an anchor (go around front of good ear first, then behind) to secure in place. If you just go around the front of the good ear with each pass, the bandage will fall down the face; if you just go behind the good ear, the bandage will fall down the neck. Obviously, do your best not to cover the pet's eyes or cause pressure to the throat when bandaging his head.
- A helpful final step is to use the sleeve off a cotton t-shirt or cut the toe off a cotton sock or thigh out of panty hose (depending on the size of the dog's head) and use as a "headband" over the ears to hold bandage in place.
- For small nicks or cuts to the ear, styptic powder may be used to control bleeding, but never use styptic powder on a deep or large wound.

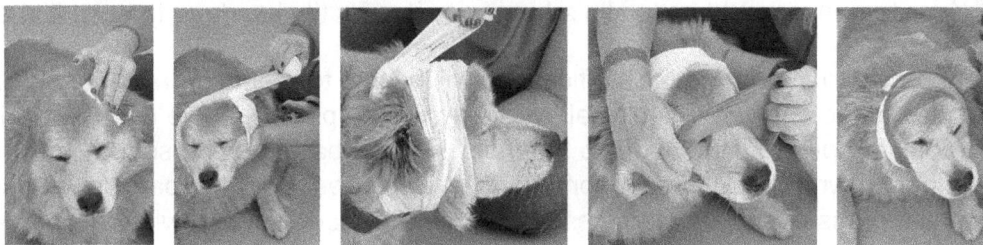

Photos by: Sunny-dog Ink

Chest Injuries

- Apply direct pressure with a flat square of gauze directly over the wound.
- There are no applicable pressure points as many blood vessels cross this area of the body.
- When applying gauze roll, wrap it around entire torso to hold in place then secure it to itself with adhesive tape. Consider only going around chest twice and then taping remaining roll of gauze onto wound to apply more direct pressure and create absorbency should wound re-start bleeding enroute to veterinary assistance.
- You can doubly secure by placing a triangular bandage under dog's chest on top of bandage and knot at back/shoulders to hold in place.
- An alternative is to fit the pet with a child's cotton t-shirt on top of the bandage or once again, depending on size of the animal, using the thigh out of panty hose, sleeve off adult t-shirt or whatever makes a snug covering. Not too tight though to limit breathing!

Important Note:

If bleeding does not stop within 5-10 minutes after applying direct pressure, seek veterinary care immediately.

144

BITES & STINGS

One Summer morning, two Dachshund pups were playfully exploring their fenced yard when Rudy caught Abigail off guard and bounded at her from behind the rose bushes. As Abby took a tumble landing dazed and confused, a bumble bee buzzed passed her. The twosome, quickly distracted by this new found fun, attempted to play a game of pounce with the tiny buzzing creature. Fun did ensue for a few moments, but it then turned nasty as the bee planted his stinger right onto the tip of Rudy's nose! The pup pawed furiously at his face, and as it began to swell, Rudy started looking more like a Bulldog than a Doxie.

CONDITION OVERVIEW:
Dogs are natural hunters and often go in search of smaller critters as prey. Just as with humans, our pets can experience an allergic or inflammatory reaction if bitten or stung. Most pets, especially dogs, are bitten or stung on the face or in the mouth since they snap at bees and other insects. Sometimes they are even stung inside their mouth but can also sit or step on a stinging insect.

PREVENTIVE MEASURES/CAUSES:
- Do your best to lessen the prey drive in your dog (using the word "no" or having a water squirt bottle nearby to deter their desire to participate in the chase), but nature will unfortunately take its course, so be prepared when the inevitable happens.
- Keep down the insect population by not leaving food outside, using pet-safe insecticides around your yard and growing plants (such as lemongrass or catnip) or lighting citronella candles (if safe around pets) that cause insects to stay away.

SIGNS & SYMPTOMS:
- Swelling
- Pawing at face or licking paws or site of sting
- Breathing difficulty -- AN EMERGENCY SITUATION

Important Note:

Anaphylactic Shock - Some dogs, like people, are highly sensitive to insect toxin and can go into Anaphylactic Shock (a severe allergic reaction which can cause the circulatory system to shut down). If you notice any of the following symptoms, which usually occur within one hour, you must seek veterinary assistance immediately:

1) Severe and profuse swelling (i.e. entire face as opposed to just the lip)
2) Difficulty breathing or increased respiratory effort possibly due to swelling of the tongue or throat.
3) Vomiting & Diarrhea
4) Very pale or blue-tinged mucous membranes (cyanosis)
5) Rapid and/or irregular pulse
6) Prolonged CRT (Capillary Refill Time) - Refer to Vitals section pages 103
7) Below normal body temperature (less than 100° F)

WHAT YOU MAY NEED:
- Cold Pack
- Baking Soda or Meat Tenderizer Containing Papain.
- Epi-pen (if your pet has had previous encounters with bees and is allergic)
- Water
- Needle-less Syringe
- Eye Dropper
- Spray Bottle
- Diphenhydramine/Benadryl® (not containing Cetirizine, Acetaminophen or Pseudoephedrine)

NOTE: If you can find liquid gel caps, pierce the cap with a straight pin and administer medicine by squirting liquid from the cap underneath the pet's tongue. The abundance of blood vessels in the mouth allows the medicine to be absorbed more quickly into the blood stream sublingually than if swallowed and processed by the stomach.

WHAT TO DO:

INSECT STINGS (Bees/Wasps):

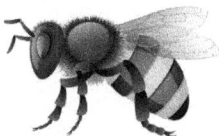

If you see the stinger, flick it away with a credit card, popsicle stick or even your finger nail. Do not pull the stinger with your fingers or tweezers as you are likely to puncture the poison sac allowing the toxin to enter the animal's body. Often though there is no stinger to be found as it is concealed in the dog's fur or has already been pawed away.

Administer 1 mg Diphenhydramine (Benadryl® antihistamine) for every pound your dog weighs (ex: 60 lbs. dog needs 60 mg). Although this medication is generally safe, check with your Veterinarian especially if your pet is taking other medications or has any known medical conditions. It will make your canine sleepy and hopefully prevent him from further scratching. Diphenhydramine should not contain cetirizine, acetaminophen or pseudoephedrine. This dose can be repeated in 6-8 hours if swelling persists. Beyond that, seek veterinary care.

Apply cold pack to any swelling, but remove every few minutes to avoid frostbite. You can also squeeze out a wet washcloth till it is just damp and place it between the cold pack and the dog to dissipate coldness.

Should you actually be able to see through your dog's fur and locate the sting site, dab it with a paste made of 1 Tablespoon baking soda or meat tenderizer mixed with a drop of water to counteract the acidity of the toxin (meat tenderizer and baking soda are alkaline). The tenderizer contains papain, an enzyme extract from papayas which breaks down the protein in the toxin. Diphenhydramine should not contain cetirizine, acetaminophen or pseudoephedrine. Baking soda and meat tenderizer also work for fire ant and jelly fish stings but not against snake venom while white vinegar is best for wasp stings.

If you have an epi-pen prescribed specifically for your dog, read attached instructions but inject one dose and get to your Veterinarian as when the epinephrine wears off, anaphylaxis can occur.

HOMEOPATHIC TIP:

Apis Meliffica, can aid the body to reduce burning or stinging pain. A dose is considered to be 3-5 pellets crushed or liquefied with 6c being given every 4-6 hours.

IF INSECT STING IS IN THE MOUTH:
- Offer pet an ice cube, frozen slice of banana or ice water to minimize swelling.
- Seek immediate advice from your veterinary professional as toxins in the mucous membranes of the mouth and under the tongue more quickly absorb into the dog's blood stream and should his tongue swell, a Veterinarian is best equipped to help.
- Call your Veterinarian as you are on the way to find out if you should administer 1mg Diphenhydramine for every pound the dog weighs or if you should wait till you arrive at the Animal Hospital.

SCORPIONS

From human experience, we know the pain from a scorpion sting can be intense. When stung, most pets recover without difficulty, however some do have a more severe reaction. There are over 1,200 different species of scorpions in the world and their venom varies with most potent enough to kill an insect or small animals, but some deadly to larger animals and humans. Scorpions can control the amount of venom injected, and those with large thick tails and slender pinchers are generally more harmful.

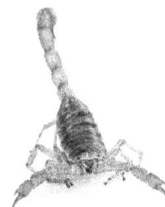

PREVENTIVE MEASURES/CAUSES:
- Do not allow dogs to roam in areas that are known to have venomous scorpions. Especially when temperatures climb above 100°F, Scorpions like damp areas around wood piles, flower beds with wood chips and plumbing fixtures, so make sure your pet can't access these areas.
- Deter scorpions from entering your home by repairing holes in window screens and adding weather stripping and caulk to seal any holes scorpions might enter through.
- Prune trees and shrubbery from near the house.
- The use of cedar oil may repel scorpions or if a problem, investigate pet-safe insecticides.

SIGNS & SYMPTOMS:
- Localized pain and/or numbness, But more severe include:
  - Drooling
  - Tearing from the eyes
  - Inappropriate urination and defecation (loss of control of bodily functions)
  - Dilated pupils
  - Muscle tremors
  - Breathing difficulty
  - Collapse

WHAT YOU MAY NEED:
- A calm you to transport your dog to the Veterinarian for assessment.
- Dead scorpion for identification if you can obtain safely.

WHAT TO DO:
Carefully remove the stinger from your canine patient if at all possible, but prompt veterinary care is strongly recommended where supportive treatment (fluids and pain medications) will be provided.

SPIDERS

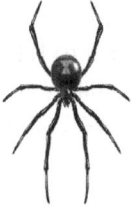

With over 30,000 species in the world, spiders exist everywhere! Most spider bites however cause little more than painful swelling and should be treated like bee or wasp stings since most spiders are unable to penetrate human or animal skin. There are a few species in the U.S. however, and more throughout the world that are venomous (inject toxin through fangs) and in addition to inflicting a painful bite, can cause our pets to experience serious side effects within 30 minutes to several hours of being stung.

In the United States, these include: Widow (5 species), Brown Recluse and Hobo spiders. The most dangerous arachnids around the world include: Brazilian Wandering, Six-Eyed Sand, Sidney Funnel Web, Redback, Mouse and Yellow Sac spiders. If your dog is bitten by one of these, get immediate veterinary help!

PREVENTIVE MEASURES/CAUSES:
- Use pet-safe insecticides to keep your house and yard spider-free.
- Clear debris piles and leaves from locations your pets hang out.
- Prevent dogs from sniffing under and around sheds, foundations, basements and damp areas, including where hoses are stored, near water spigots and leaky plumbing -- basically cool, dark, damp locations.

SIGNS & SYMPTOMS:
- Swelling/Redness
- Licking at or rubbing area of the sting
- In severe cases...pain, fever, rash, chills, breathing difficulty, vomiting, diarrhea, lethargy, muscle tremors or rigidness, paralysis (including of the lungs) and shock

WHAT YOU MAY NEED:
- Benadryl® (not containing Cetirizine, Acetaminophen or Pseudoephedrine)
- Baking Soda or Meat Tenderizer
- Water
- Cold Pack

WHAT TO DO:
As in Bee Stings already discussed, Administer 1 mg Diphenhydramine (Benadryl® antihistamine) for every pound your dog weighs (ex: 60 lbs. dog needs 60 mg). Benadryl® should not contain cetirizine, Acetaminophen or pseudoephedrine and do not give pets time release capsules. See Allergy page 130 for more details. Spider toxin also contains acid, so applying an alkaline baking soda or meat tenderizer paste (as described in BEE STINGS) may counteract the acidity.

Apply cold pack to any swelling, but remove every few minutes to avoid frostbite.

If you suspect your dog has been bitten by a venomous spider, apply a cold pack, restrain his movement (movement hastens the spread of venom) and get him quickly to your Veterinarian. If you can, bring the dead spider with you unless you already know what kind of spider it was.

Black Widow Spiders terrify us all with their distinctive red hour-glass marking (some are brown with orange hour glasses, mostly in Florida but they travel). About ½" - 1" long (1.2cm - 2.54 cm) they prefer warm, dry climates and spin their webs in crevices and protected dark locations. Both the male and female Black Widow possess a nerve toxin, but only the female has long enough fangs to penetrate a dog's skin. If you could find the bite under the animal's fur, you may note a slight redness with two small puncture wounds 1-2mm apart. Muscle cramps, pain, increased heart rate, vomiting, diarrhea and paralysis follow. Small dogs may experience more severe effects due to the venom ratio to their smaller body size, but location of the bite, health and age of the pooch and even time of the year (venom is thought to be more potent during warmer times of year) all play a role. If you suspect a bite, have your Veterinarian evaluate your dog immediately. Antivenin is available with mixed results but pain medications and muscle relaxants may help pull your dog through.

Brown Recluse (aka Fiddleback) Spiders tend to hide in dark, secluded areas and their venom is known to destroy tissue (necrosis) surrounding the bite. Approximately ½" - 2" long (1.2cm - 5cm), the Brown Recluse can be identified by a distinctive fiddle-shaped mark on its back. Generally found in the South Central U.S. (Texas through Georgia) they are being found elsewhere. When bitten, most dogs do not realize it, but after a while redness occurs often in the shape of a bulls-eye which is generally not noticeable on our dogs. Seek veterinary assistance at once. Animals are treated with pain medications and antibiotics and some wounds require surgical closure.

Hobo or Travelling Spiders can destroy your dog's tissue with their bite. Found mostly in the Pacific Northwest, these large and aggressive brown spiders (often confused with the Recluse) build their webs in basements or at ground level. If a bite is suspected, get your dog to the Veterinarian!

Many **Tarantulas** are furry exotic pets but some species found in the U.S. produce venom that can cause localized pain. Not only can the mild venom cause problems for your dog, but also the ingestion of the stiff hair covering the spider's legs can cause irritation to your pet's mouth including pain, drooling and vomiting. Tarantula's can actually "flick" hairs at targets when threatened, so don't allow dog's to get too close. If your pet is bitten, no serious problems should be expected but it is always best to err on the side of caution and have your Veterinarian check Fido out. On the reverse…the jumping nature of your eight-legged pet Tarantula makes it an irresistible plaything to many four-legged pets, and a Tarantula can die from a bite caused by a dog.

Fly Bites or Fly Strikes

CONDITION OVERVIEW:

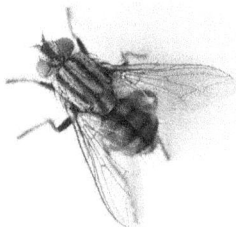

Dogs with upright ears seem to hold the biggest temptation for flies but the bridge of the nose or any body part where skin is visible can be bitten. The Stable Fly – which looks like a regular House Fly – has bayonet-like, needle-sharp mouthparts which it uses to get blood from your pet. Dogs with fly bites don't bleed much but the ear tips get crusty from inflammation and the serum that leaks from the bites. Fly bites leave bloody lumps on your pet and in the worst cases, lay eggs from which maggots can hatch.

PREVENTIVE MEASURES/CAUSES:

- Remove items that attract flies: pick up pet feces daily, cover garbage cans, pick up fallen fruit
- Place fly traps in strategic locations if this is a serious problem
- Bring your dog inside, especially during warm weather when flies congregate most
- Apply petroleum jelly or Avon® Skin-so-Soft lotion on the tips of your pet's ears to deter flies
- Add 1 Tablespoon Apple Cider Vinegar to your dog's water -- some people swear flies won't bite an animal or human who drinks Apple Cider Vinegar!

WHAT YOU MAY NEED:

- Chlorhexidine or mild soap
- Triple Antibiotic Cream (Neosporin®-type product)
- Warm, wet washcloth or gauze squares

WHAT TO DO:

Soften the scab with a warm wet washcloth. Take 2-3 minutes until it can be gently wiped away.

Clean with an antiseptic liquid soap like Betadine® or Chlorhexidine. For cats, plain warm water is safest.

Apply an antibiotic ointment to prevent infection and keep your dogs fly-free.

If your pup must be outside, consult with your Veterinarian in regards to a topical fly repellant that can be applied to your canine.

If wounds won't heal or you see any presence of maggots, get your dog to professional veterinary help!

CONDITION OVERVIEW:

Another danger to our furry friends comes in the form of venomous and non-venomous snakes. Yes, even those without venom (toxic saliva) carry bacteria in their mouths (they don't brush their teeth and consume rats and mice on a daily basis) which can cause infection in your dog. The physical appearance of each snake species varies, and it may be difficult to tell which species you've encountered unless you are familiar with herpetology (the study of amphibians and reptiles).

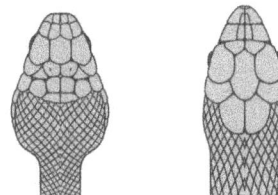

Here are general guidelines to help you determine if what you are seeing is a poisonous snake although there are always exceptions to the rule:

- A broad, triangular head with a noticeable "neck"
- Vertical slits like cats for pupils while non-venomous snakes generally have round pupils like us and our dogs (hopefully you won't be close enough to evaluate this!)
- "Pit vipers" have heat-sensing "pits" (thermo-receptors) on their faces between the eye and nostril which help them locate prey, especially warm-blooded animals.
- Two fangs which leave puncture wounds. Non-venomous snakes leave a bite or bruise mark that resembles a row of teeth – like when you bite out of a sandwich but much smaller.
- In the case of the rattlesnake, a rattle is present which may or may not issue a warning.

Rattles are made of keratin, similar to our fingernails. When a baby snake is born, he has one button/segment of his rattle. Each time he sheds his skin, he acquires another segment (shedding typically occurs several times a year based on food supply and growth). At least two segments are required to vibrate against each other to create a noise. If a snake has not shed his skin for the first time he will not be able to rattle. Snakes generally carry their rattles high to protect them, they do break from time to time. Although rattles are considered warning devices, some snakes have evolved into not using them as the sound wards off prey that could become a tasty meal.

Venomous snakes can be found in rural areas as well as suburban areas where there is sufficient natural habitat. In cold climates most hibernate from November through March. In warmer climates, however they are active year round, and after mild winters, they come out of hibernation early.

Follow the WHAT TO DO steps below for any of these venomous snakes and get your pet to the Veterinarian immediately!

- Rattlesnakes can be found throughout most of the south from California to Florida.
- Copperheads live mostly in North Florida to Massachusetts and westward to Texas and Nebraska.
- Cottonmouths/Water moccasins inhabit Illinois, Missouri, Oklahoma and Texas north east to Virginia and south to Florida. As a rule, venomous water snakes typically keep their entire bodies above water, while non-venomous remain submerged except for their heads.
- Coral snakes are typically found in the Southeast (Texas to Florida) and have tri-colored bands of red, yellow and black that completely encircle the body. "Red touching yellow is a dangerous fellow" as opposed to the "red touching black, venom he lacks" scarlet king snake which is non-venomous. King snakes in other parts of the country are colored differently.

Learn which species are indigenous to your neighborhood as well as to any locations you may travel to with your pet. The list above is only a guideline, so just like you must know your pet, you need to know what local dangers he may encounter BEFORE he does so!

Most snakes can control the amount of venom they inject and often deliver a "dry" bite to a human or large animal. Baby snakes, however, are born with venom and the means to inject it but aren't yet "fang trained," so generally hold on longer and deliver all the venom they have at one time. Older snakes possess more potent venom and larger snakes store larger volumes of it.

This toxic fluid, made from up to 25 different enzymes, comes in two forms created in specialized oral glands: Hemotoxic venom disrupts the integrity of the blood vessels causing swelling as blood seeps into the tissue and prevents clotting. It also breaks down the tissue and "pre-digests" it making it easier for the snake to consume. Neurotoxic venom results in paralysis including that of the respiratory muscles ending in suffocation. Some snakes possess both types.

The degree of severity of any venomous snake bite depends on several factors:
- The species & size of snake
- The size of the animal bitten
- The amount of venom injected (approximately 20% of bites are "dry" meaning envenomation has not occurred, but that means 80% of the time it has!)

PREVENTIVE MEASURES/CAUSES:

- As with many other scenarios requiring pet first-aid, prevention is key, so your best safety device is keeping control of the animals in your care. It is easier to prevent snake bites than it is to treat them.
- Keep dogs on-leash when hiking so that you can steer them clear of dangerous critters.
- Stick to open paths as heavily travelled areas are less likely inhabited by reptiles.
- Don't let pets sniff under rocks and logs (yeah, but it's where snakes hide out)! Do your best to step ON fallen logs rather than over them to cover holes underneath and prevent the snake from striking as you and your dog step over.
- Eliminate garbage, wood piles and even ivy from pet play areas. These are favorite locales of mice, and where mice hang out...snakes line up for dinner! Look into a rattlesnake aversion class to see if it can lessen the prey drive in dogs eager to go on the chase. These classes are offered in many areas and train dogs to recognize the sight, sound and smell of a snake. In a short 15-20 minute lesson (often renewed annually), dogs are taught to steer clear of snakes by the use of a remote training collar. Seek a course in your area that offers positive reinforcement to train your best pal.

SIGNS & SYMPTOMS:

- Puncture wounds ("U" shaped bite or bruise if non-venomous)
- Drooling
- Shortness of breath
- Swelling
- Diarrhea
- Seizures/convulsions
- Inability to bark
- Paralysis
- Shock

WHAT YOU MAY NEED:

- As in most pet first-aid...a calm you! Phone and phone number to call ahead
- Transportation to the Animal ER
- Chlorhexidine/antibacterial soap ONLY if a non-venomous bite

WHAT TO DO:
If you are certain it was a <u>non-venomous</u> snake...

Wash the wound with antibacterial soap and observe.

If red or warm to the touch, get to the Veterinarian for antibiotics or other treatment.

If an dog in your care is bitten by a snake, it is best to assume it was a <u>venomous</u> bite and proceed as follows:

- Keep bite wound below level of heart to prevent speedy absorption to heart.
- Keep animal calm – the faster he moves, the faster the venom circulates.
- Get the animal to an emergency veterinary hospital immediately to be sure they have antivenin. Treatment should begin within 30 minutes of the bite, and it takes 30 minutes to mix the antidote!

WHAT NOT TO DO:
- **Do NOT** cut over the bite and try to suck out the poison. You will not be successful and may absorb under your tongue or in any mouth sore. Additionally, by cutting tissue, you are more readily allowing toxin to be absorbed.
- **Do NOT** manipulate the bitten area or allow the dog to move about freely.
- **Do NOT** place an ice pack over the bite. This will concentrate the toxin more locally causing extensive, irreparable tissue damage.

Important Note:
Antivenin is an antidote: a serum produced to neutralize the effects of the venom. In laboratories, healthy horses are injected with increasing amounts (non-fatal) of selected snake venom causing the horse to create antibodies from which the antivenin is made. A specific antibody is produced for each type of snake (typically four different crotaline/rattlesnakes). Antivenin is reconstituted before use and given to your furry patient via an IV drip that takes 30+ minutes per vial. It is expensive ($800 - $1,500 per vial) and although a large dog is likely to require 3-4 vials, some many require up to 10 vials to save their lives, plus antibiotics, fluids and pain medications to see him through. Antivenin is only currently available for certain species of snakes. Dogs bitten by other species are treated for symptoms presented. This just underscores the importance of avoidance training and diligent supervision if you frequent or live in areas that are common for venomous snakes.

Rattlesnake Vaccine is not a cure-all but can minimize the severity, which has the two-fold benefit of giving more time (before death occurs) to get to a Veterinarian and may reduce the number of antivenin vials needed for treatment. For these reasons, the vaccination is beneficial if you live in a snake-prone area. Check with your Veterinarian for details.

Jelly Fish Stings

CONDITION OVERVIEW:

Jelly fish are extraordinary yet simple marine animals characterized by their jelly-like bodies and stinging tentacles. Among the oldest creatures on earth, there are around 10,000 different species and they get their proper name "cnidarians" from the Greek word for "sea nettle." When they come in contact with prey -- meaning you or your dog – their tentacles literally explode causing great pain

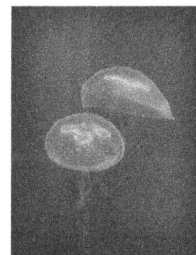

PREVENTIVE MEASURES/CAUSES:
- Avoid high risk areas when visiting the beach with your dog by:
    - Looking for warning signs – diamond shape informational signs that depict a human and a jelly fish.
    - Noticing purple flags which denote dangerous marine life.
    - Keep your dog on leash and away from the water's edge during windy times. Jelly fish come near shore when it is windy and show up in large numbers (known as blooms).
    - Do not touch or let your pet anywhere near a jelly fish, even if it appears dead. Poisonous cells on dead jelly fish can still sting! They often look like plastic bags, bluish-purple bottles or light bulbs. Keep a watchful eye and keep your dog out of harm's way.

WHAT YOU MAY NEED:
- Rubbing alcohol or white vinegar
- Rubber Gloves
- Stick tape - any kind but NOT duct tape
- Benadryl® (not containing Cetirizine, Acetaminophen or Pseudoephedrine)
- Baking Soda
- Ice pack

WHAT TO DO:

Put on rubber gloves or you will be stung too, and pour rubbing alcohol or white vinegar onto the tentacles. This stabilizes the namtocysts preventing them from continuing to sting your dog. Next take small sections of sticky tape (like for packing boxes) and gently press against tentacle, pull tape away to remove. Once you've done a good clean-up of the tentacles, flush the affected area with salt water or even beach sand. Fresh water will cause toxins to be released into your dog! Call your Veterinarian and you may be advised to administer Benedryl® (1mg per pound of your pet's body weight). Packing the site of the sting with a baking soda/water paste may soothe the pain as can a cold compress. After 10 - 20 minutes, alternate every 5 minutes with a very warm (but not scalding) towel. Remove and let it cool to bring healing blood back to the area flushing out the toxin. Then reapply the cold compress followed by the warm towel for about 20 minutes or until veterinary care is reached.

Bloat (Gastric Dilatation & Volvulus or GDV)

CONDITION OVERVIEW:

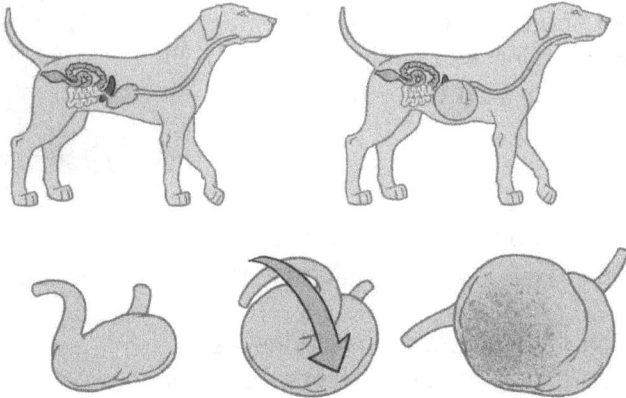

The proper medical term for bloat is gastric-dilatation-volvulus (GDV) which means that your dog's stomach has become overstretched and may have twisted. This is a very serious condition that can have fatal results in as little as 10 – 20 minutes so immediate veterinary treatment is needed!

As your dog's stomach becomes enlarged (or bloated) with food, fluid and/or gas, it can rotate 90-360° which decreases blood flow to and from the heart as well as to organs below the stomach. This leads to shock, abnormal heart rhythms and decreased oxygen to all tissues of the body. Treatment involves correction of shock as well as emergency surgery to de-rotate the stomach and empty its contents. Depending on the severity and duration of the GDV, portions of the stomach may become necrotic (tissue death) and need to be removed. The most important part of the surgery is to permanently attach the stomach to the body wall (gastropexy) to prevent future twisting of the stomach because once a dog has bloated…it is likely to happen again.

Bloat mostly occurs when dogs consume large quantities of food or swallow excess air while eating but can also occur when the valve at the bottom of the stomach becomes blocked and gas or other material produced by the digestive process can't exit the stomach.

Although exact causes of bloat aren't always determined, a pet's breed, age and genetics are believed to play a prime role. Large deep-chested breeds are more prone to bloating and if there is a family history (60% increased chance if parent or sibling has suffered bloat) or if the dog is an older, underweight male he too is at higher risk. Stress may also play a role.

PREVENTIVE MEASURES/CAUSES:

- Exercise – After meals a potty break is always advisable, and a casual stroll is actually encouraged, but no running, swimming, chasing a ball, rolling in the grass or even fast walking for 1 ½ - 2 hours after food is consumed. A full belly can swing like a pendulum during brisk movement and flip. On the reverse, if your dog has been exercising, always wait until his respiration is back to a normal resting rate before feeding or allowing him to drink from his water bowl.
- Gulping food – When a dog eats fast he swallows large chunks and excess air, both of which can quickly fill the stomach. Slow down a voracious appetite by using one of the tips below advising smaller meals, specialized bowls or even toys for feeding.
- Smaller meals – The twice daily feedings may help in another way as many dogs who eat one large meal weigh down the stomach stretching out their hepatogastric ligament. The job of this ligament is to keep the stomach in its proper position in the abdomen, so if it weakens or extends, the stomach may rotate.
- Raised bowls – Many believe feeding a large dog at a raised dog table prevents the ingestion of excess air but others feel dogs may consume food more quickly from a raised feeder since they don't need to stop and lift head occasionally to swallow. Currently there is much discussion so please confer with your Veterinarian and/or breeder as to the pros and cons, and observe your dog to ascertain what is best for him.
- Specialty Bowls – Slowing down the consumption of food may also prevent air gulping which could lead to bloat. Many bowls are now on the market that have obstacles for your pet to eat around. Another idea is to feed your dog by placing his meal in a toy that makes him work for it, getting only small bits at a time.
- Kibble – Providing a moisture-rich diet by adding canned or other wet food to the kibble may reduce the risk of bloat. Some experts debate whether water consumption prior to mealtime may dilute gastric acids needed for proper digestion. With research ongoing, YOU, your Veterinarian and canine nutritionist are your best resources as you can personally evaluate the health of your dog. Know your dog, his breed and family history if available, seek out expert advice and stay vigilant to anything that is not normal!
- Stress – At the groomer, boarding facility, turmoil at home, long car rides, in a shelter or stress for other reasons can all contribute to bloat. Dogs with fearful and nervous personalities also have a higher incidence of bloat than their calm and relaxed counterparts.
- Preventive Surgery – High risk dogs may be candidates for a prophylactic gastropexy. This surgery can easily be performed at the same time as your pet's spay/neuter. Both procedures use a minimally invasive technique when done as a preventive and could spare Fido problems down the road.

SIGNS & SYMPTOMS:

- Distended, swollen-looking belly that appears quickly; feels hard to the touch
- Retching; may also moan in discomfort or have the dry heaves; animal tries to vomit but can only bring up ropey, foamy saliva
- May try to defecate but is unsuccessful as organs below the stomach have shut down although he may be able to in beginning stages
- Restlessness, anxious or collapse; dog displays a difficult time getting comfortable and may pace
- Difficulty breathing; red or pale blue gums
- May glance or try to bite or lick at their belly (bloat is similar to colic in horses)

BREEDS MOST SUSCEPTIBLE INCLUDE
(although it has been documented in others including small dogs):

Airdales, Akitas, Alaskan Malamutes, Basset Hounds, Bernese Mountain Dogs, Bouviers, Boxers, Chesapeake Bay, Golden & Labrador Retrievers, Collies, Doberman Pinschers, German Shepherds, Great Pyrenees, Newfoundlands, Old English Sheepdogs, Pointers, Rottweilers, Samoyeds, Setters, Spaniels, St. Bernards, Standard Poodles, Weimareners, Wolfhounds

WHAT YOU MAY NEED:

- Once again, nothing can be more helpful to your ailing dog than a pet parent who remains calm and quickly transports him to veterinary help.
- If he cannot move, a board, blanket or towel can prove helpful (See page 124 on transporting an injured pet).

WHAT TO DO:

Get to your Veterinarian ASAP. Do not delay! This is a life-threatening condition that will not correct itself. Your dog could die in as little as 10-20 minutes. Your Veterinarian needs to insert a tube into the stomach, but if twisting has occurred, emergency surgery needs to take place.

BLOOD SUGAR ISSUES -

Low (Hypoglycemia or Fading) & High (Hyperglycemia/Diabetes Mellitus)

CONDITION OVERVIEW:

Insulin, a hormone that is produced and released by the pancreas into the bloodstream when glucose levels rise, plays a key role in maintaining normal sugar levels. As it moves glucose through the body, it gives ours pets their energy for life. The normal blood sugar level for dogs and cats is 75 to 120 mg/dl (milligrams per deciliter), but the level can be as high as 250 to 300 mg/dl after a meal or in stressful situations, such as visiting the Veterinarian's office.

Hypoglycemia (aka low blood sugar) occurs when levels drop below 60 mg/dl. It primarily occurs in our tiniest four-legged friends, including Toy breeds and juvenile animals (less than 4 months of age). Very active adult dogs, however, may experience low sugar if sustained exercise has caused a depletion in liver glycogen (sugar).

When not enough insulin is produced hyperglycemia is the outcome and your dog may be diagnosed with diabetes mellitus if sugar levels exceed 400mg/dl. This means conscientious dog parenting is a must as a lifetime of treatment is in store for your pet, starting with insulin injections and a special diet to keep the sugars in check.

PREVENTIVE MEASURES/CAUSES FOR HYPOGLYCEMIA (low blood sugar):

- Annual check-ups and blood tests as suggested by your Veterinarian can alert you to a problem.
- Susceptible pets should be fed small amounts frequently throughout the day of a high quality protein and fiber/low sugar, carbohydrate and fat diet as instructed by your Veterinarian. This will help keep glucose levels constant. Also, check if adding a tablespoon of Karo® Syrup to your pet's daily drinking water would be beneficial for at-risk pets. If you do so though, you MUST change the water EVERY day as the sugar can grow bacteria (You are however changing the water and washing the bowl daily anyway with warm soapy water, right? It's an important part of good pet parenting!).
- Extremely active pets should receive high quality protein before exhibiting long bouts of energy, but of course with a lengthy digestion period in between to prevent bloat..
- Keep any product containing xylitol out of paws reach as it causes an increase in insulin which can drop your pet's glucose level in 30 minutes to 12 hours after ingestion. Read labels on sugar-free sweeteners, gums and candies, certain jams and baking products, over–the–counter and prescription medications and dental hygiene products as well as anything you suspect your pet could ingest that could contain xylitol or anything labeled "sugar alcohols". Veterinary treatment is key as liver failure can result.

SIGNS & SYMPTOMS FOR HYPOGLYCEMIA (low blood sugar):
- Twitching, shaking or wooziness; disorientation as if they are intoxicated
- Weakness/lethargy
- Head tilt
- Seizures
- Loss of consciousness

This is serious. Dogs can die without quick first-aid and medical attention if diabetic!

WHAT YOU MAY NEED FOR HYPOGLYCEMIA (low blood sugar):
- Karo® or Pancake Syrup
- Honey
- Needle-less Syringe or Eye Dropper
- Blanket

WHAT TO DO FOR HYPOGLYCEMIA (low blood sugar):
The quickest way to reverse hypoglycemia is to administer sugar by mouth (honey, Karo Syrup®, pancake syrup) –
- 1 teaspoon for pets under 50 lbs.
- 2 teaspoons for animals 50 - 80 lbs.
- 2 ½ - 3 teaspoons for extra-large breeds.

If dog is unconscious or can't swallow, rub the syrup on the lips and gums. If animal is not alert and breathing normally, treat for shock (See page 213 to increase circulation and cover to keep in body heat) as you seek immediate veterinary attention. Watch for breathing and check for pulse and administer rescue breathing and/or CPR if needed.

PREVENTIVE MEASURES/CAUSES FOR HYPERGLYCEMIA (high blood sugar):
- Avoid high intake of sugar in your dog's diet.
- Don't miss annual check-ups or let infections go unchecked.

SIGNS & SYMPTOMS FOR HYPERGLYCEMIA (high blood sugar):
- Increased thirst and/or hunger
- Increased urination
- Weight loss or weight gain
- Dehydration
- Cataracts and/or inflamed blood vessels in the eyes
- Enlarged Liver
- Open sores that won't heal
- Nerve damage in limbs

WHAT YOU MAY NEED FOR HYPERGLYCEMIA (high blood sugar):
- Prescribed medication and syringe (see page 113 for details on giving injections, but learning in person from your Veterinarian is best).

WHAT TO DO FOR HYPERGLYCEMIA (high blood sugar):
Once diagnosed, diabetic dogs can live a wonderful life with human caretakers as long as life-long compliance is maintained to properly manage the disease. Urine and ear prick testing with an at-home glucometer can help keep your Fido's glucose levels in check.

If insulin has been prescribed, correct dosing is a must at the right time of day. Too much, not enough or a too soon or delayed dose can be very dangerous for your furry friend. Additionally, a special low sugar and low carbohydrate diet with higher protein and fiber may be recommended. It is imperative that you strictly follow treatment guidelines for the health of your canine patient and friend.

BURNS

CONDITION OVERVIEW:
Just like in humans, the skin is your dog's largest organ, and serious injury can happen to it. Heat, chemicals and electrical sources can all be the cause. Second and third degree burns are highly susceptible to infection since many layers of tissue have been destroyed. A visit to your Veterinarian is in order, but cooling the skin is essential and should be done slowly over a 30-minute period.

PREVENTIVE MEASURES/CAUSES:
- Be aware of ever-present dangers...when you have a dog, you have an inquisitive furry toddler for life.
- Beware when removing pots and pans from still-hot burners by preventing your pooch from jumping up, and never pass hot plates or liquids over your pet's head. Also, think twice about stepping over dogs, especially with anything in your hands, as it is Murphy's Law that when you step over your dog will stand up!
- Candles, even on countertops, can be toppled by or burn dogs who jump up high.
- Outdoor cook-outs are tempting to Fido, so never turn your back while food is cooking or even when it isn't as the smell coming from hot coals and grills lasts a long time.
- Supervise dogs around fire pits/camp fires, fireplaces and heat sources of all types -- electric heaters, furnaces, hot pavement, even beach sand during the peak of summer.
- Too much sun can burn the muzzle, ear tips, back or belly, especially on breeds without a thick undercoat. A shorter summer trim is fine but never shave your pet as fur protects his skin from the harsh sun.
- Beach sand, sidewalks and asphalt can burn paws...if you can't walk on it barefoot, it's too hot for your pets!
- Anything hot to the touch -- if you could get burned, so could your dog!

First Degree Burns

SIGNS & SYMPTOMS:
Skin appears pink to dark pink or red (usually sunburn on the snout, ears or belly skin), could be slightly swollen

WHAT YOU MAY NEED:
- Room Temperature Water
- Cold Pack
- Aloe Vera Gel or Triple Antibiotic Cream
- Soft Cloth or Gauze
- Blunt-Nosed Scissors

NOTE: Thermal burns start out sterile as heat kills bacteria. Take care not to contaminate wounds by trying to "clean" or cover with non-sterile materials.

WHAT TO DO:
The first goal is to cool the pink skin with room temperature water (not ice water which restricts circulation).

Pat dry and apply pure aloe vera gel to promote healing after carefully trimming fur away with blunt-nosed scissors.

If skin is unbroken, home care should suffice by holding a cold pack (not ice) over the wound for another 20 minutes and observing that it heals while preventing your pet from obsessive licking or scratching the injured area.

Second Degree Burns

SIGNS & SYMPTOMS:
- Pink to red skin with the presence of blisters and/or serous fluid (aka pus)
- Extremely painful & susceptible to infection as tissue damage has occurred

WHAT YOU MAY NEED:
- Muzzle
- Room Temperature Water
- Soft Cloth
- Non-stick/Teflon Coated Gauze Pad
- Gauze Roll or Clean White Sheet to Cover
- Adhesive Tape to Secure Loose Bandage

WHAT TO DO:
Get to your Veterinarian but call first! Intravenous fluids, antibiotics and hospitalization may be needed.

Calmly and quickly, first check respiration, pulse and treat for signs of shock (see page 213).

Safely muzzle pet if no breathing difficulties are present as even the gentlest dog could bite when enduring great pain.

Flush gently with or immerse burned areas in cool (not ice) water while you are checking on the phone with your Veterinarian for further instructions. Burns can continue to cause damage even after the initial source of the burn has been removed. The flow of cool water reduces temperature below the skin surface to help prevent further damage, but it must be done slowly over a period of time rather than taking quick measures with ice which could lower your dog's body temperature or add frostbite to the injuries.

Pat dry with a soft cloth (not cotton balls which leave fibers behind).

Bandage loosely (or wrap in a clean sheet but use non-stick pad closest to burn if possible) to keep clean and prevent anything from entering damaged tissue and seek veterinary help immediately.

DO NOT apply any gels, ointments or sprays until seen by a Veterinarian.

If no infection occurs, healing can occur as quickly as 3 weeks.

Third Degree Burns

SIGNS & SYMPTOMS:
- Surface of the skin will appear charred, white or leathery and brown (An unpleasant visual, but think black like a charred burger you left on the grill too long; white like a boiled chicken breast. Your pet's tissue has in fact cooked!)
- Swelling under the skin or absence of skin.
- Third degree burns go through all the layers of skin and into the muscle underneath.
- Pain, although sometimes due to the destruction of nerve endings, is not immediately as painful as 2nd degree burns.

WHAT YOU MAY NEED:
- Muzzle
- Room Temperature Water
- Non-Stick Gauze
- Gauze Rolls
- Adhesive Tape
- Clean White Sheet or Other Smooth Fabric

WHAT TO DO:
Seek immediate veterinary care but call first!

Intravenous fluids, antibiotics and hospitalization may be needed.

Calmly and quickly, first check respiration, pulse and treat for signs of shock (see page 213).

Safely muzzle if no breathing difficulties are present as an animal in severe pain may bite.

Flush gently with or immerse burned areas in cool (not ice) water while you are checking on the phone with your Veterinarian for further instructions. Burns can continue to cause damage even after the initial source of the burn has been removed. The flow of cool water reduces temperature below the skin surface to help preventfurther damage but it must be done slowly over a period of time rather than taking quick measures with ice which could lower your pet's body temperature or add frostbite to the injuries.

Pat dry with a soft cloth (not cotton balls which leave fibers behind).

Bandage (or wrap in a clean sheet but use non-stick pad closest to burn if possible) to keep clean and prevent anything from entering damaged tissue and seek veterinary help immediately.

DO NOT apply any gels, ointments or sprays until seen by a Veterinarian.

During transport to the veterinary facility, monitor the animal for signs of shock (see page 213).

Chemical Burns

SIGNS & SYMPTOMS:
- Can exhibit signs of first, second or third degree burns (see previous pages) with the addition of a foreign substance (chemical) on the fur or skin.

WHAT YOU MAY NEED:
- Room Temperature Water
- Liquid Dish Soap or Shampoo
- Cold Pack
- Aloe Vera Gel or Triple Antibiotic Cream
- Non-Stick Gauze
- Gauze Rolls
- Adhesive Tape
- Clean White Sheet or Other Smooth Fabric
- Blunt-nosed Scissors
- Disposable Gloves for You
- Goggles or Eye Protection

WHAT TO DO:
Protect yourself first, if you are injured then you are no help to your dog. Put on disposable gloves and use protective eyewear in case the animal shakes or the chemical you are removing splashes into your eyes or on to your skin.

If available, read chemical label for appropriate treatment. Otherwise, flush liquid chemicals from pet's body with large amounts of room temperature water for at least 10 minutes (water that is too hot may speed up the absorption of the chemical through the skin while water that is too cold can cause hypothermia).

- If you believe that an animal in your care has been exposed to a chemical agent that may affect their lungs, seek veterinary care immediately.
- If chemical is oily/greasy, gently massage dishwashing liquid into the fur/skin first to dissolve grease before flushing with water. Take care as if the chemical has reached skin, your dog may be sore to the touch.
- If it is a dry chemical (powdered or granular), brush away or even vacuum out of the animal's fur if he will allow you to do so safely. Adding water may further activate the chemical so do not flush with water until any dry chemical has been removed. This even applies to laundry soap which is easier to remove in bulk while dry than when it lathers. Lathered soaps may also be strong and burn your dog's skin, so brush away first.
- Seek veterinary assistance immediately if the burn appears to be second or third degree (as described on page 162).
- Bring the chemical container (if possible) with you to the veterinary facility in a zip lock bag or by other safe method of transport.

Electrical Burns

CONDITION OVERVIEW:
A dog who receives an electric shock may have burns and/or the shock may cause an irregular heartbeat resulting in cardiac arrest. Damage may also occur to the capillaries in the lungs leading to fluid accumulation (pulmonary edema) causing respiratory difficulties or failure.

Do not touch an animal that is/has been electrocuted until the electricity (circuit breaker) is off or the source of electrocution (wires) has been safely moved away with a non-conducive material such as wood or plastic.

PREVENTIVE MEASURES/CAUSES:
- Place cords in locations inaccessible to dogs or unplug when not in use
- Use outlet covers
- Cover cords with plastic sleeves or special tubing
- Teach dogs NOT to chew and provide other appropriate chewing activities for teething puppies

SIGNS & SYMPTOMS:
- Unconscious
- Belabored breathing
- Visible burns or wounds
- Bite marks on an electrical cord or a burning odor in the room could imply your dog was burned or received a shock

WHAT YOU MAY NEED:
- Gauze Squares, Rolls & Adhesive Tape or Flexible Wrap
- Non-Conductive stick to move away electrical wires

WHAT TO DO:

Immediately check if the dog is breathing and has a pulse.

If the dog is not breathing, administer rescue breathing or CPCR (if heartbeat is also absent) and get to your Veterinarian immediately.

Even if the dog is conscious after electrocution, it is still advisable to seek veterinary attention because even minor electrical shocks can damage blood vessels in the lungs which could cause a slow leak of fluid that can make breathing difficult. It can take any where from several hours to a few days before symptoms (shortness of breath, loss of appetite, lethargy) set in. Do not delay veterinary care.

Check the animal for burns to the face or in the mouth, and provide wound treatment (See Bleeding Injuries page 140).

BUMPS & LUMPS

CONDITION OVERVIEW:

Lumps are often a concern – they are easy to feel and make pet parents think something is wrong with their furry child. Lumps are divided into two groups:

- Benign – Non-cancerous lumps may grow bigger but do not spread elsewhere.

- Malignant - Aggressive cancerous lumps which not only grow but also spread through the body and may affect vital organs.

The most common lumps are lipomas (benign fatty tumors), papillomas (wart-like growths or tags) and sebaceous cysts (which often drain a creamy fluid). Sometimes benign lumps are removed as they can be a nuisance if they continue to grow by restricting the movement of a leg or joint, pressing on the airway or other organs.

Mammary tumors can appear on both males and females and should be removed, but if found early, may not be problematic.

Mast cell tumors can be benign but are most often malignant and should generally be removed before they spread to other areas of the body.

PREVENTIVE MEASURES/CAUSES:
- Read labels on products used around your dog
- Dose flea repellants and other medications properly
- Perform weekly head-to-tail check-ups to find trouble spots early
- Don't skip annual veterinary visits
- Talk to your Veterinarian about titer tests before getting annual vaccinations
- Provide a nutritious diet with high quality protein, no fillers, food colorings or cancer causing preservatives

SIGNS & SYMPTOMS:

- Abnormal swellings that persist or continue to grow
- Sores that won't heal
- Weight loss
- Loss of appetite, difficulty eating or swallowing
- Bleeding or discharge from any opening on the body
- Offensive odor
- Reluctance to exercise or tires quickly
- Lameness or stiffness that won't go away
- Difficulty breathing, urinating or defecating

If you suspect anything is "not quite right" with your dog, it is best to have your medical professional check him out immediately.

WHAT YOU MAY NEED:

- Veterinary appointment

WHAT TO DO:

Follow veterinary instructions

Many things can cause a lump – bruising, swelling caused by fluid build-up, hematomas (blood filled sacs), abscesses (sacs of pus often near puncture wounds), ticks, foxtails or any protrusion. You can't tell just by looking at it even if you are a Veterinarian! However, there are several clues that may help your vet decide whether a lump on your dog is likely to be benign or malignant:

- If the lump moves (i.e., if it can be picked up in the fingers and moved around), it is less likely to be aggressive, **but only your Veterinarian can tell for sure**.

- If the lump is firm, fast growing and does not move, it is more likely to be malignant as these lumps grow into the tissue below the skin, **but only your Veterinarian can tell for sure**.

If the lump is red, painful when touched or is discharging fluid and if your pet seems to not be feeling well, get it checked out immediately. Testing a lump can be as easy as putting a needle into it to collect a few cells or your Veterinarian may feel it is necessary to take a piece of the lump under anesthesia to best determine what kind of lump it is. Once the type is known, your Veterinarian will be able to advise you on the best treatment for your pet.

One in every three dogs will suffer from cancer making it the number one killer of dogs over two years of age. When certain canine cancers are discovered early, the probability of a positive outcome can be good. Every year advances are made in canine cancer research, so do those head-to-tail check-ups weekly and don't miss an annual visit to your Veterinarian!

Cancer Primer

Hemangiosarcoma is most commonly found in the spleen, liver and heart. Prognosis is determined by location of the disease.

Adenocarcinomas present in the anal sacs on either side of the rectum. Size can range greatly and symptoms vary depending upon gender of the pet but can include increased thirst, weakness, persistent licking at the site, difficulty defecating and decreased appetite.

Lymphoma is cancer of the lymphatic tissue which is a core part of the body's immune system. The most common sign is a painless enlargement of the lymph nodes.

Mast cell tumors are among the most common tumors found in dogs generally found on the skin, spleen, liver and bone marrow but contain chemicals that can be released into surrounding tissue. They vary greatly in size, shape, appearance and texture. The only way to definitively identify is through a biopsy.

Osteosarcoma is the most common bone tumor in dogs but can spread throughout the blood stream early on (metastasis). Frequently, it's found in the wrist, shoulder, knee and hip. Lameness due to pain followed by swelling are first signs.

Sarcomas Soft tissue sarcomas are a group of several different types of tumors made of connective tissue (bone, muscle, joint). They are located either within the skin, or in tissues just below the skin so are often discovered when petting or grooming your furry friend.

Squamous cell carcinoma occurs in the mouth, under the tongue and along the gum line in middle-aged and older pets. Common signs include difficulty eating, drooling and odor from the mouth.

Transitional cell carcinoma tumors usually form at the bladder opening causing painful urination. Pets often strain or may have blood in the urine making it difficult to diagnose since these are the same symptoms for urinary tract infections, which often delays diagnosis.

CLOTHES DRYER INJURIES

CONDITION OVERVIEW:
Burns, broken bones, abrasions, heat stroke, breathing/suffocation and cardiac arrest can occur when a small dog curls up in a warm clothes dryer to sleep, and his unwary owner throws a load of clothes on top of him and starts the dryer.

PREVENTIVE MEASURES/CAUSES:
- Make it a habit to keep the washer and dryer closed when not in use, and always check inside before using. Follow the same practice with refrigerators and freezers. Although more of a feline incident, small dogs too are curious… are curious creatures and they can quickly jump into one of those appliances when your back is turned. Be diligent when you have a four-legged "toddler" and make sure his environment is safe.

SIGNS & SYMPTOMS:
- Burns/Singed fur
- Redness, pain, wounds/abrasions
- Broken bones
- Cardiac and/or pulmonary arrest

WHAT YOU MAY NEED:
- Teflon Coated Gauze Squares
- Gauze Rolls
- Water
- Splinting Materials (popsicle sticks, unsharpened pencils, wooden spoons, rolled up magazines, bubble wrap, to name just a few, in addition to an actual Sam Splint®)

WHAT TO DO:
Check if dog is conscious and breathing. If not, immediately administer CPR. If dog is alert, treat according to injuries (cool burns with water), splint or place on back board if you suspect broken bones and get to the Veterinarian immediately.

CONSTIPATION

CONDITION OVERVIEW:
Difficult or infrequent bowel movements are painful and hazardous to your dog. Healthy pets have 1-2 stools per day so a day or two without is a cause for concern. When an animal is constipated, toxins remain in the body.

PREVENTIVE MEASURES/CAUSES:
- Pay attention to your pets and monitor bathroom habits. You won't know if your dog is relieving himself if you let him run stray in the neighborhood. Walk your dog or notice if he's answering nature's call in your fenced yard.
- Do not give dogs cooked bones, which not only can puncture but can also block the intestines.
- Monitor dogs around toys and notice if articles of clothing are missing -- in other words, keep items that might tempt your dog out of paws reach.
- Make sure dogs are provided a diet with some fiber and plenty of fresh water at all times.

SIGNS & SYMPTOMS:
- Dog is straining to go with no results or crying in pain
- Hard stools, possibly covered with mucous or blood
- Lethargy
- Vomiting
- Abdominal discomfort
- Dehydration
- Enlarged colon
- Arthritis
- Hypothyroidism (thyroid deficiency)

WHAT YOU NEED:
- Sugar-Free Bran Cereal
- Canned Pumpkin Puree * (not pumpkin pie mix which has added sugars and ingredients)

*TIP: When opening a can of pumpkin, spoon left-overs into an ice cube tray and freeze. Then pop frozen 1 tablespoon servings into a zip lock bag and keep in the freezer until next time. Dehydrated varieties are also available so that you may mix up only as much as needed and some contain apple fiber which also aids in elimination.

WHAT TO DO:
If this is a first time occurrence, try one of the following methods of relief:
- Keep your dog well hydrated by encouraging water consumption.
- Feed 1 tablespoon sugar-free bran cereal for a small dog and up to 3 tablespoons for a large dog; check with your Veterinarian but Metamucil®-type wafers are often a good choice.
- The authors' personal favorite home remedy is to feed pureed cooked pumpkin! Give 1 tablespoon to a cat or small dog and up to 3 tablespoons for a large dog.

Most pets like the smooth texture and the fiber pushes things through the colon! If animal has not resumed normal bowel movements in 24 hours, seek veterinary care.

COUGHING

CONDITION OVERVIEW:
Coughing is a reflex resulting from an irritation in the airway. People cough to eliminate dust, bacteria and itchy things from our throats and windpipes, but for pets coughing is unusual. While coughing up the occasional hairball isn't anything to worry about, coughing that lasts a day or more could be the sign of a respiratory infection, bronchitis, or congestive heart failure, so don't delay in getting your pet to the Veterinarian!

PREVENTIVE MEASURES/CAUSES:
- Adjust collars and leashes so that they don't restrict the trachea.
- Observe pets while they are eating and playing with toys to make sure they don't become choking obstructions.
- Take notice of chemical, fumes, and foods that might be irritating your pet.
- At the first sign of distress in your dog, have him checked out by his medical professional.

SIGNS & SYMPTOMS:
- Wet/moist cough could indicate fluid or phlegm in the lungs.
- Choking cough, with pawing at mouth could mean the pet is choking (page 129) or collar is too tight.
- Do not smoke in the presence of your dogs as they can develop emphysema from second-hand smoke.
- Observe your dog's reaction to aerosol sprays, cleaners, fertilizers and chemicals of any type used around your house and yard. Many will irritate your pet resulting in coughing or breathing difficulties.
- Dry/hacking cough, worsened by exercise or excitement, could mean kennel cough.
- Dry cough with spitting up saliva only could mean bloat (page 156) -- check for distended abdomen! Gagging cough, followed by lip licking and swallowing, could be symptomatic of an infection. Prolonged coughing at night or while lying down could suggest heart disease.
- A "goose-honk" cough, especially in toy breeds, could indicate a collapsing trachea.

WHAT YOU MAY NEED:
- A calm demeanor to check throat for obstructions or loosen collar
- Humidifier
- Honey
- Lemon
- Water

WHAT TO DO:

Take collar off. An irritated airway will benefit from less pressure being placed on it. Instead use a harness to keep your pet safe.

If your pet is experiencing a dry cough, humidify the air or sit with him in the bathroom while you run the shower to moisten up the room and his airway.

Administer a natural cough syrup! Dogs love 2 tablespoons honey mixed with1 teaspoon of lemon in a ½ cup of water. Give it to your pooch twice daily or more frequently if needed – 1 tablespoon for 50 lbs.or more dogs and 1 teaspoon for your smaller dogs.

A wonderful herb that can prove helpful in eliminating coughing and fluid build-up is Dandelion. The leaves have a diuretic property, that removes excess fluid from the body. Find a quality health food store and give 2 drops per pound of your pet's body weight of the tincture twice daily.

If the cough lasts more than a day or two, take your pet to the Veterinarian as it could be serious or at least require additional meds. Don't purchase OTC cough syrups without veterinary advice as many contain acetaminophen, aspirin or other hidden ingredients. Two homeopathic remedies your Veterinarian may suggest are *Belladona* for a dry cough and *Pulsatilla* for a cough that is dry at night and loose (productive meaning fluid is being coughed up) in the morning.

CPCR (CARDIO PULMONARY CEREBRAL RESUSCITATION)

Please refer to page 122 in this handbook.

DEAFNESS

CONDITION OVERVIEW:
Are doorbells and electric can openers no longer getting a rise out of your dog? Do you find your dog is easily startled when you enter a room? For an animal to hear sounds, cells that transmit vibrations as well as the brains cells that interpret them, must be intact and functioning properly.

Birth defects, disease, injury and even medication can cause animals to lose hearing. A Veterinarian can assess and determine the correct course of action, but don't lose heart… pets are remarkably adaptable and can often hear something if you find the right pitch. Fido may no longer hear those low mellow tones, but he might be able to discern a higher pitch if used to call his name.

PREVENTIVE MEASURES/CAUSES:
- Always check your dog's ears for foxtails and other debris after walks and hikes.
- Place a large cotton ball in your pet's ears when bathing to avoid fluid build-up and fungal infections. Keep your dog's ears free of wax which can block the ear canals, but never use a cotton swab as you could damage the ear drum.
- Only use medications as prescribed.

SIGNS & SYMPTOMS:
- No longer obeys commands, seems to wander aimlessly or looks confused.
- Dogs with predominantly white coats (Dalmatians for instance) and ones with Merle patterns (marbled such as some Shelties and Australian Cattledogs/Blue Heelers) are at higher risk for deafness due to a lack of pigment in the "hair cells" that detect sound. About 60 breeds are prone to genetic deafness, but if these dogs have pigmented cells in the inner ear, they usually can hear normally. Additionally, having blue eyes also increases the risk for deafness with the non-hearing ear often found on the same side as the blue eye.

WHAT YOU MAY NEED:
- Your hands! Clap behind dog to see if there is a response.
- Whistle or other noise makers to test your pet's range of hearing.

WHAT TO DO:
Veterinary check-up where your pet professional can assess cause and degree of deafness and determine if any medical treatments are an option.

Help your precious pet adjust to a new yet good quality life…
- Always walk your dog on a leash and keep him out of harm's way in a safely fenced yard.
- Teach him signals: "Come" by waving your hand towards yourself or flicking the kitchen light switch on and off for instance.

- Gently stomp your feet when you approach so as not to startle your dog. Owners sometimes believe their dog has late on-set aggression when in fact he is just startled by someone he didn't hear coming. Approach deaf dogs head-on, so that you are seen, and create vibrations so that they won't be caught off guard and nip to protect themselves.
- Get your four-legged friend a four-legged companion whose cues he can follow to know when someone is at the door.
- Most important of all, however, is to be patient with your best friend who is going through a transition and needs your continued love and support.

DEHYDRATION

CONDITION OVERVIEW:
Dehydration can be fatal as water is essential to all living beings! It makes up 3/4 of your pet's body and aids in circulation, digestion and the elimination of toxins. When your dog is over-heated from exercise or temperature, or when he is ill and suffering from vomiting or diarrhea, he can lose up to 10% of his body weight quickly through fluid loss. Elderly, pregnant or nursing pets and ones with diabetes are most prone to dehydration.

PREVENTIVE MEASURES/CAUSES:
- Hydrate, hydrate, hydrate! Always make sure your dog has plenty of cool fresh water available and monitor his drinking habits…he should consume about 1 ounce of water for every pound he weighs daily! Keep your toilet lid closed so that he'll drink from a bacteria-free source and make sure his water bowl is washed daily with warm soap and water and never goes dry.
- Tune in to your dog so as to alert to increased body temperature, runny stools or even constipation (which could imply inadequate fluid intake).
- Endocrine diseases such as Addison's and diabetes can contribute.

SIGNS & SYMPTOMS:
- Gums feel dry or sticky to the touch.
- Tugor Test -- Skin stays in a "tent" or falls back in place slowly rather than snapping back when you gently pull up on it over your pet's neck, upper back or even on the top of his head in the case of looser-skinned breeds such as Basset Hounds and Shar Peis.
- Sunken eyes
- Lethargy
- Loss of appetite
- Depression
- Delayed Capillary Refill Time

<u>**WHAT YOU MAY NEED:**</u>
- Needle-less Syringe, Eye Dropper, Turkey Baster or even clean spray bottle with water
- Electrolyte Solution (pet brands exist or make your own below)
  - 1 Quart Fresh Water (bottled or filtered preferred)
  - 1 Tablespoon Honey
  - 1 Teaspoon Salt

Mix and store in refrigerator but serve at room temperature making a fresh batch daily. Throughout the day, dose:

- 3 Tablespoons for puppies/kittens
- 5 Tablespoons for pets up to 5 lbs.
- 3/4 cups for pets up to 10 lbs.
- 1/4 cup per 5 lbs. of body weight for pets 15 lbs. and more

To keep on hand, mix 4 cups water with 1 teaspoon salt and 1 teaspoon sugar and freeze in ice cube trays.

<u>**WHAT TO DO:**</u>
If dog's temperature is normal (100.4°F – 102.5° F) encourage him to drink or offer him some electrolyte solution. If temperature is higher, dribble small amounts of solution through a syringe onto tongue or spray small amount of water into mouth. Forcing an over-heated dog to drink could cause him to vomit and possibly aspirate into his lungs. Dogs with a temperature 104° F or higher MUST see a Veterinarian and receive subcutaneous fluids. Dehydration can be very serious!

DIABETES

<u>**CONDITION OVERVIEW**</u>:
Is your dog thirstier than usual or eating more? Is he asking for more potty breaks or even having accidents? Just like humans, pets produce a hormone called insulin that enables their cells to secrete glucose which is used as fuel. Animals with diabetes either don't produce enough insulin or the insulin they do make doesn't work efficiently meaning their cells do not get the fuel they need. Obesity, pancreatitis, hyperthyroidism and poisons can contribute to this condition. Also see Blood Sugar Issues on page 159.

<u>**PREVENTIVE MEASURES/CAUSES**</u>:
- Get annual check-ups at your Veterinarian and at the sign of increased thirst or urination.
- Don't overfeed sugary items to your pet.

<u>**SIGNS & SYMPTOMS**</u>:
- Increased thirst and urination
- Unusually sweet breath

<u>**In later stages**</u>:
- Loss of appetite
- Vomiting
- Lethargy and Coma
- Cataracts in dogs

<u>**WHAT YOU MAY NEED**</u>:
- Insulin as prescribed.
- Honey or Karo® Syrup
- Appropriate diet

<u>**WHAT TO DO**</u>:
Have your Veterinarian confirm diabetes through blood and urine testing.

Follow prescribed regime of insulin injections or other medications. Stay on schedule!

Keep your pet at a healthy weight and well exercised.

Feed smaller meals more frequently to keep blood sugar at an even keel and switch to a high-fiber diet if recommended by your dog's health care provider.

Giving insulin can sometimes cause blood sugar to plummet (hypoglycemia) so with a diabetic dog, always have honey or Karo® Syrup on hand to rub on your dog's gums should he suddenly get shaky. (See LOW BLOOD SUGAR page 159).

DIARRHEA & VOMITING

CONDITION OVERVIEW:

Although vomiting and diarrhea are both common signs of many poisons and illnesses, most often they are caused by simple digestive upsets -- your pet ate too much, too fast or something that was spoiled like out of the garbage can. Items ranging from moldy bread to rotten apples can upset your pet's stomach. Frequent loose or liquid bowel movements can come on quickly and last only a brief period of time. Ongoing bouts of diarrhea, however, can lead to dehydration and may indicate an underlying health concern. Pay attention to your dog's bodily habits. Monitor your dog on walks or in your fenced backyard to stay on top of their health and well-being.

Knowing the difference between vomiting and regurgitation can help your Veterinarian evaluate what is up with your pooch. Vomiting occurs when food or liquid, is expelled from your pet's stomach or upper small intestine and is generally preceded by audible retching. If it originated in the stomach, it may include clear liquid while yellow or green liquid clues you in that it came from the small intestine. Of course undigested or partially digested food may also come forth.

Regurgitation differs in that the expelled material almost always comes from the esophagus (the muscular tube that propels water, food and saliva downward into the stomach). When your dog regurgitates, he brings up water, saliva and undigested food silently and the suddenness of it takes you both by surprise. A concern though is that since it occurs quickly, the larynx (opening to the windpipe) often doesn't have time to close and some of the regurgitated matter can be inhaled into the lungs resulting in aspiration pneumonia.

PREVENTIVE MEASURES/CAUSES:

- Regularly get down on all fours and check your house and yard for items your dog might get into or even absorb through his paws, and do your doggone best to keep dangers out of paws reach!
- Prevent your dog from drinking water from lakes, streams, out of gutters, buckets and unsanitary sources. Wash his water bowl with warm water and soap daily.
- Don't feed table scraps (fat, grease, salts or rich foods) or change your dog's diet suddenly.
- Ensure dogs are eating slowly (not gulping un-chewed chunks) and if a problem, slow them down with special designed bowls, providing smaller amounts more frequently or feeding from toys in which they have to work for their food and can't swallow it all at once.
- Reduce stress in your pet's life as well as in your own.
- Provide regular check-ups making sure titers are high (see page 49) or vaccines are up-to-date so that your pets won't contract disease.

SIGNS & SYMPTOMS:
- Loose or frequent stools sometimes containing blood mucus
- Flatulence
- Straining or urgency to go
- Weight loss
- Dehydration
- Fever
- Lethargy
- Vomiting

WHAT YOU MAY NEED:
- Antacid
- Syringe or tablespoon to measure
- Electrolytes
- Plenty of fresh water
- Pumpkin Puree * (not pumpkin pie mix which has added sugars and ingredients)
- Ginger Snap Cookies, Ginger Root or Capsules

WHAT TO DO:
If an animal in your care is experiencing vomiting and/or diarrhea and you know that it is not the result of poisoning:
- Rest the stomach by withholding food for 24 hours but always provide fresh water to prevent dehydration. Pedialyte® (diluted 50/50 with water) or a dog-specific electrolyte replenisher (see recipe for homemade version on page 174) can replace minerals taken out of the body due to diarrhea or vomiting.
- Administer antacid every 4-6 hours...Pepcid®, Tums® or Mylanta® are good choices. In liquid form the dose is 1 teaspoon for every 10-15 lbs. your dog weighs. Although fine for most humans, avoid Pepto-Bismol® and any products containing salicylic acid which can be harmful to your pet. Gaviscon® works too, just note the strength it comes in and do not use for dogs with kidney disease due to high level of magnesium. 15 - 45 ml/per kg of pet's weight, so ... if 5ml = 1 teaspoon and 1lbs. = 2.2 kg and you have 64 mg/ml strength of Gaviscon®, a 45 lbs. dog would get 1 - 3 teaspoons.
- Pumpkin puree is a beneficial natural cure as most animals like the taste and the fiber helps firm up loose stools. Dose 1 tablespoon for small dogs and up to 3 tablespoons for a large dog.
- Ginger! Ginger snap cookies (human kind are usually the easiest to dose and can also cure an upset tummy.) Two cookies for a medium-sized dog generally does the trick. As for pure ginger capsules...100 mg for every 25 lbs. your pet weighs repeated every 6-8 hours, or if Fido or Fluffy will drink, peel fresh ginger root, make 5-8 ¼" thick slices and boil in ¼ cup water. When it cools, let him lap it up. Any of these ginger tips may also work if administered 20-30 minutes before a road trip to keep motion sickness at bay.
- If all is well in 24 hours, you probably have a hungry canine on your hands so feed a bland diet for a few days (plain steamed rice and boiled white chicken is a good option) before getting your dog back on his regular diet.

- If vomiting/diarrhea persist beyond 24 hours, or if at any time you notice blood, get to your Veterinarian and bring a vomit/diarrhea sample along.

HOMEOPATHIC TIPS: For gastrointestinal distress or even pancreatitis, along with veterinary care, *Nux Vomica* (commonly known as Strychnine Tree) given 2x daily can help. For diarrhea, *Arsenicum Album* (1 30c tablet per 20 lbs. of body weight every 4 hours) is a good choice or Phosphorous if there is blood in the stool such as with colitis. Incorporating western herbs such as *Slippery Elm* (500 mg 2X daily for a large dog) can aid with Irritable Bowel Syndrome, Diarrhea and Constipation while aloe vera is beneficial for gas and acid reflux – dried form is better tolerated by animals than the gel. Additionally, chamomile or peppermint can be made into a tea to settle tummies and rehydrate. Give 1 tablespoon for every 10 lbs. your pet weighs repeating every 4-6 hours.

DROWNING

CONDITION OVERVIEW:

Drowning occurs when there is an accumulation of fluid in the lungs, typically when an animal is immersed in a body of water but it can also occur on dry land when fluid is aspirated into the lungs. With water in the lungs, there is no room for oxygen and suffocation occurs. Submersion time, water temperature as well as whether it was fresh, salt or chemical water will affect the prognosis. Some pets recover from near drowning incidents only to develop fluid in the lungs (pulmonary edema) hours later. Known as "dry drowning," this too can be fatal so anytime your pet has fallen into water, have him checked out by your veterinary professional at once! Also see Water Toxicity (page 221).

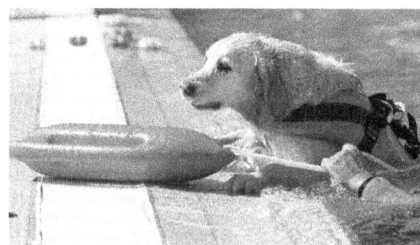

PREVENTIVE MEASURES/CAUSES:
- Not all dogs know how to swim – it's not an innate trait even for so-called water dogs! Dogs with short necks have a particularly difficult time keeping their heads above water. Make any water environment safe for Fido and Fluffy by fencing it off, attaching a pet ramp to the side of swimming pools or making dogs wear a life-jacket when at the lake or boating. Even good swimmers tire, and since they can't rest with paws on the bottom nor tread water, a jacket can help keep them afloat.
- Refresh those dogs that swim each season as to where the way out of the pool is!
- Keep your eyes on your pets at all times when they are near the water. Accidents only take seconds to occur. Your dog could fatigue while swimming, your dog could fall through ice, get caught in a flood, suffer a head injury or seizure while in or near the water.
- Never force water into an animal trying to make him drink. Administer slowly with a needle-less syringe or eye dropper when trying to hydrate.

SIGNS & SYMPTOMS:

- There is little guesswork involved in this injury. If you find an animal in a body of water, get them out!
- Blue gums/skins
- Coughing with clear to red foam
- Crackling sound from the chest
- Unconscious to barely conscious
- Difficulty breathing or absence of breathing and pulse

WHAT YOU MAY NEED:

- Towel, rope, life preserver, long pole -- something to help you get dog out of the water but if he is conscious and struggling, take appropriate measures so that they do not pull you under
- Cushions, folded towels to elevate hind quarters on larger animals
- Towels, blankets to warm pet in
- Karo Syrup® or Honey
- Calm demeanor to perform necessary tasks to help your best friend
- Transportation to veterinary help

WHAT TO DO:

Quickly remove the dog from water. If he is struggling, it is best for you not to enter but rather stay near shore or pool side so that he won't pull you under in his state of panic.

Hold small dogs securely by the hind legs to drain water from lungs, windpipe and mouth. For larger dogs, place in wheelbarrow position (front legs on ground while you hold up hind legs) taking care not to hit snout or head of unconscious animal on ground. If this method is unsafe for the handler or is unsuccessful, lay the dog on his side and elevate hind quarters with cushions to help drain water. With the animal on his side, it may help release water if you place the heel of your hand in the dip behind the last rib and thrust up sharply towards the head 3-4 times. Do not spend more than a few seconds doing this however since the lungs quickly absorb water and any water that does not come out quickly probably won't come out at all.

If you detect a heartbeat but the dog is not breathing, begin rescue breathing immediately. Wrap the animal in towels or blankets to keep from going into hypothermia and continue rescue breathing until the animal shows signs of recovery or until a veterinary professional can take over. Oddly enough, research has shown that water 90° F and below can slow the rate at which brain cells die, so some animals that have spent a considerable time in cold water have a good chance at recovery.

If the dog is not breathing and a heartbeat is absent, begin CPCR and get prompt veterinary attention. Do not stop CPCR unless the animal shows signs of recovery or until a veterinary professional can take over. If you have additional hands, rub Karo ® Syrup or honey on the dog's gums which could aid in resuscitation.

Even when you are lucky enough to revive Fido, immediately follow-up with a veterinary visit for assessment of any life-threatening inflammation to the lungs.

EMBEDDED OBJECTS

CONDITION OVERVIEW:

Due to their inquisitive nature and scavenging habits, our pets are likely to get a foreign object embedded in their skin. Glass, thorns, needles and sticks are most common, but could include an arrow or quill from a porcupine. Removing an object that is penetrating deeply could result in massive blood loss and tissue damage, so first aid may include securing it in place and acquiring immediate medical attention.

PREVENTIVE MEASURES/CAUSES:

- Keep your yard clear of dangers and watch as you walk through parks and on trails with your dog for shining glass, bramble or anything that could puncture paws or any body part.
- Monitor dogs around lakes where there could be fishhooks or other sharp objects.
- Take special care in places like garages and workshops where many small but sharp items can be easily dropped.
- Don't allow dogs near locations where bow & arrow shooting may occur.

WHAT YOU MAY NEED:

- Gauze squares & rolls
- Adhesive tape or flexible wrap
- Tweezers
- Paper or Styrofoam cup; empty margarine tub
- Disposable gloves
- Scissors
- Saline solution or purified water to clean
- Triple antibiotic cream
- Towel or board to carry injured dog to transportation

WHAT TO DO:

If you find an animal in the unfortunate situation of having a stick, arrow or other object embedded in a body part:

- Keep the dog as still as possible. Remember that like many other times first aid is in order, you may need to restrain and muzzle the animal (see page 109).
- If it is a small object and doesn't appear to be too deeply embedded, remove with tweezers, clean and bandage (see page 140).
- If object is large or deep in skin and area is bleeding externally, secure the object in the exact position it is in by placing gauze rolls on each side and wrapping with a third roll.
- Make this wrap snug enough to hold the object in place but not tight enough to restrict blood flow or breathing. The idea is to secure the object so that it won't move and cause further tissue damage while you are transporting the cat or dog to the Veterinarian. You can also make a ring bandage by first tying a triangular bandage into a tiny loop, and then wrapping each of the "tails" around the loop to form a ring. Finally tying those ends together and placing ring around imbedded object to keep it in place.
- An alternative would be to brace the imbedded object in place by cutting a hole in the top or slit the side of a plastic margarine tub or Styrofoam cup – the slit allows the object to penetrate up and through the container but remain still. Then tape the

container firmly to the pet's body to prevent movement as removing objects sometimes cause great loss of blood so it is best done under professional medical care.
- Do not attempt to brace or stabilize an imbedded object if the animal is struggling, resistant or showing obvious signs of extreme pain and/or aggression. The dog could either cause the object to become imbedded further or cause physical harm to you (the first-responder).
- Transport the dog to the veterinary hospital immediately.

EYE INJURIES

CONDITION OVERVIEW:
A variety of eye issues can befall our four-legged friends: scratches to the cornea, cherry eye (oval pink mass of flesh protruding from the eye), entropion (portion of the eyelid is inverted or folded inward irritating the cornea), prolapse (eye comes out of socket) or blood-filled eye due to rupture of capillaries (subjunctive hematoma). With the exception of a speck of dirt or debris which can be flushed away, these injuries are best dealt with at your Veterinarian's office. As our dogs age (and sometimes earlier) cloudiness or hardening of the cornea develops. Once again, your veterinary professional is key to helping your dog maintain sufficient vision and comfort.

PREVENTIVE MEASURES/CAUSES:
- Take note of toys your dog plays with – stiff nylon whiskers and other sharp parts should be cut off of stuffed animals so as not to scratch your dog's eye when he chews on them.
- Observe your dog anytime he rubs his eye on the ground or with his paw. Tiny claws from other animals may scratch (raccoons are the most vicious). Running through hedges which are nothing but small sticks and possible sharp leaves can also cause damage to delicate corneal tissue. Catch problems early and have your Veterinarian care for in a timely manner.
- Upper respiratory infections and other illnesses can cause redness, swelling and even prolapse so know your dog to quickly identify anything that is not quite right.

SIGNS & SYMPTOMS:
- Redness, pawing at the eye, rapid blinking, swelling
- Excessive tearing or any discharge
- Clouded cornea (the front clear covering of the eye)
- Unequally dilated pupils or lack of response of pupils could be a medical emergency

WHAT YOU MAY NEED:
- Eye Wash (Saline or Purified Water)
- Gauze squares
- Non-stick Gauze if covering eye
- Adhesive tape or flexible wrap

WHAT TO DO:

Cleanse the eye with sterile eye wash by pulling upwards on top lid to open eye wide and flushing from outer corner of eye making sure extra fluid and debris run down muzzle. Let dog blink out extra liquid. Inspect in good light to make sure the foreign object has been removed.

If the eye is out of the socket or blood is present, cover with non-stick gauze dampened with eye wash and get to professional help immediately.

Do not attempt to pull ANYTHING that is penetrating eye ball. If it does not flush away, bandage in place (without applying additional pressure) and get quickly to your Veterinarian!

FALLS & HIGH RISE SYNDROME

CONDITION OVERVIEW:

Although most of us think of feline companions as being the species up in high places, dogs are even more likely to be injured in the event of a fall. Their bodies are denser than a cat's and dogs do not generally right themselves which means they fall faster and harder, exponentially increasing the likelihood of severe injury. Many are injured from falls, so take care to prevent the worst from happening to your canine friend. From a fall out a window, off of a balcony, off a piece of furniture or a high place, dogs can sustain a variety of injuries including broken bones, jaws, ruptured organs and even death. If you notice your dog is limping or refusing to move or eat, it is possible that your dog could have suffered an internal injury that may not be easily noticed but can become dangerous very quickly.

PREVENTIVE MEASURES/CAUSES:

- Make sure you have screens securely in place on all windows and don't give dogs unsupervised access to balconies, rooftops or other high places.
- Some dogs are climbers. Even if you don't live in "earthquake country," secure shelves, bookcases, television sets and anything that your canine pal might climb upon so that it can't fall when he jumps up.
- Don't place dogs in harm's way for photo ops or other reasons. Four on the floor on sturdy ground is best!

SIGNS & SYMPTOMS:

Head Injuries:
- Confused/unstable
- Blood or clear cerebral spinal fluid coming out of ears, nose and/or eyes
- One pupil larger or pupils non-reactive to light

Spinal Injuries:
- Unstable, crooked stance of head/neck or paralysis
- Breathing & bleeding concerns

- Gauze squares and gauze rolls
- Adhesive tape or flexible wrap
- Towel, board, cookie sheet (and strips of fabric to restrain animal to board) to move or lift pet
- Muzzle

WHAT TO DO:

Check to see if your dog is breathing. If not, administer rescue breathing by giving two quick breaths into his nose while closing his mouth. Make sure the chest rises. Then give breaths according to chart on page 124 until pet breathes on his own or you reach medical help.

Every 30 seconds, check for a pulse at her inner thigh (femoral artery) or by cupping your hand behind the front elbow at the chest feeling for heart beat. If there is none, begin CPCR (see pages 122). Do realize though, this is not a cure, and you must quickly get your dog to the Veterinarian even if he starts breathing on his own. Transport the dog so as to cause little disturbance to his body (on an improvised backboard) and secure him with rolled gauze or stronger material (even a leash may do) so that he does not shift off of it.

If your dog is breathing, check for bleeding injuries. Apply direct pressure with a sterile gauze pad to stop external bleeding and prevent infection. If you notice a "sucking" chest wound (you'll see bubbling and hear air rushing into the body as your cat strains to breathe), wrap his body with plastic wrap to seal it and get your dog to the Veterinarian immediately -- do not delay. See Bleeding Injuries, Rescue Breathing, CPCR and Transporting an Injured Animal sections of this book for further details.

Realize any blood coming from or pooling in the eyes, nose or mouth could mean a head injury or internal bleeding requiring quick medical attention. Don't forget that a conscious pooch in pain may bite even his most loyal human friend, so restrain his head with a towel or use a muzzle as long as it doesn't interfere with injuries.

FROSTBITE

CONDITION OVERVIEW:

Animals don't tell us when their paws get numb. We find out only when it hurts for them to step or when we notice tissue has become hard and dark. Frostbite is a condition that can occur as a result of exposure to freezing or subfreezing temperatures. It most commonly affects the tips of the ears, the tail, the scrotum and the paws, especially the toes. When your four-legged best friend is in a cold environment, their body responds by reducing blood flow to the extreme parts of their body. This provides good blood flow to their vital organs but decreases the oxygen and warmth in the extremities allowing ice crystals to form in the tissue.

Near Chagrin Falls, Ohio, a white Maltese named Beau went out his doggie door during a blizzard to answer nature's call. The eight-year-old 13 lbs. pooch did not quickly return, and his owner found him outside looking like a white statue. According to Beau's Veterinarian,

Dr. Carol Osborne, "We quickly wrapped him to warm his body, assessed his vitals and discovered his heart rate was low as was his body temperature of 98° F!" The staff blew his wet coat dry, gave him warm subcutaneous (under the skin) fluids and a vitamin injection. Osborne adds, "Beau was offered warm chicken noodle soup and recovered just fine."

All dogs aren't so lucky. Although frostbite is not the same as hypothermia (when a canine's body temperature drops and stays below the normal range of 100.4° F – 102.5° F), a dog can experience both when he remains in the cold. He can end up with patches of frostbitten skin as well as damage to the internal organs and often cannot be saved. Medication for heart conditions and diabetes may increase risk as do windy conditions, if the dog gets wet or if he is a senior.

PREVENTIVE MEASURES/CAUSES:
- Use common sense and limit time outdoors. When hiking, periodically warm ear flaps between your hands, check paws to keep snow and ice from between the toes and never let your faithful friend out in the winter without accompanying her.
- Short furred dogs without under coats can benefit from a dog sweater when outside for even short periods of time.
- A temperature of 10° F or below is too cold for a dog to withstand, but there are just too many variables to predict at what temperature tissue damage will occur. Arctic breeds usually do better than Chihuahuas and the length and thickness of coat, a dog's age, other health issues, conditioning to the cold, wind chill and dampness all play a role.
- If your dog must remain outdoors, well-insulated dry bedding is a must for winter (straw is a popular choice). Outdoor dogs caloric intake should be increased by at least 25% to generate the necessary body heat that could be lost during colder days, but…not so fast for indoor dogs who probably exercise less and could pack on the pounds.
- Watch for hard tissue varying in color from pale to gray as this could mean frostbite and may not be detected unless the fur has sloughed off. Once the area defrosts, the skin will redden and become tender. In severe cases, the tissue turns black within a few days and dies.

WHAT YOU MAY NEED:
- Towels, blanket
- Clothes dryer
- Warm liquids and syringe to administer if they won't lap it up

WHAT TO DO:
Wrap frozen paws with blankets (tumbled briefly in a warm — not hot — clothes dryer) but do not massage area if tissue is hard as it will hurt. Never use a heating pad or hot water bottle as you may damage nerves and blood vessels.

Lower effected area (legs, paw, tail) by having pet lie in your lap or on a sofa to promote circulation to frostbitten parts.

Seek veterinary assistance immediately. As the tissue warms, frostbite turns painful, and Veterinarian Brooks Bloomfield of Truckee-Tahoe sadly explains, "Many of the dogs I've seen had accelerated heart rates due to pain and some self-mutilated their paws and tail as the circulation returned." Therefore, veterinary care is imperative. Additionally, antibiotics may be prescribed to prevent infection along with pain relief medication. In severe cases, amputation or surgical removal of affected tissue is not uncommon, so do all you can to keep your dog from becoming a canine icicle and help him live a longer, happier, healthier life with you!

HEAD ENTRAPMENT

CONDITION OVERVIEW:
Fido chases Fluffy or reaches his head through a fence or gate only to find out that what went through will not come back out!

PREVENTIVE MEASURES/CAUSES:
- Examine your house and yard for fences, spaces between walls, pool equipment, work benches and any place your dog can get stuck or a body part trapped. Dogs can outsmart us, but the more you pay attention to your environment from your dog's point of view, the more likely you are to see a possible accident waiting to happen.

SIGNS & SYMPTOMS:
- Head is stuck in a gate or fence and the dog cannot move.

WHAT YOU MAY NEED:
- Patience and calming vibes to share with your pet
- Petroleum or K-Y® Jelly, baby oil or any type of grease to help slip your dog's head back through the barrier

WHAT TO DO:
Call your Animal Ambulance Service if needed, but first and foremost…stay calm and keep your dog calm as well. Rapid movements and jerking about can cause great damage to his head and neck. Stand close to your dog, preferably positioning yourself behind him and holding his body close to what he is trapped in so as not to strain his neck by pulling on it. If he isn't having trouble breathing, muzzling might be a good idea to protect yourself.

Once he's relaxed, use a lubricant like K-Y or petroleum jelly to grease the fur of his neck and especially the crest of his skull (the thickest part of the head) as well as the bars/fencing that he is stuck in (even baby oil will work). This will help him slide and keep the fence rail or other object from scraping skin as the dog's head comes free. Your dog's head most likely is narrower from top to bottom than it is from side to side, so you can often free a trapped dog by gently turning his head sideways.

If that isn't working and the bars or obstacle can be pried apart without causing pressure to the dog's head or neck, that would be an appropriate Plan B.

Provide follow-up care to any cuts or scrapes and if you fear there has been any neck or spinal injury, do not hesitate...get to your Veterinarian for x-rays.

When all is well, come up with a solution so that your pet can not become entrapped again.

HEAD PRESSING

CONDITION OVERVIEW:
The compulsive act of a dog pressing his head against a solid surface for extended periods of time. It generally indicates a nervous system problem or neurological illness or condition and should be evaluated by your Veterinarian at once.

PREVENTIVE MEASURES/CAUSES:
- Head Trauma
- Tumors or damage to the brain or skull including encephalitis
- Stroke
- Metabolic Disorder (Hyper or Hyponatremia – too much or too little sodium in the body's blood plasma)
- Toxic Poisoning
- Liver Disease
- Infection of the Nervous System (Rabies, Parasites, Bacterial, Fungal or Viral)

SIGNS & SYMPTOMS:
- Standing or lying with forehead pressed against a wall, sofa or other solid surface or pushing head into the ground
- Pacing or walking in circles
- Getting stuck in corners
- Staring at walls
- Visual problems
- Seizures
- Reflexes not functioning appropriately

WHAT YOU MAY NEED:
- Safe transport to the Veterinarian for diagnosis.

WHAT TO DO:
By recognizing the signs and getting an immediate veterinary evaluation, you just might save your dog's life.

HEAD SHAKING

CONDITION OVERVIEW:
When it comes to canines, any itch, sting or irritation may prompt them to shake their head in hopes of getting rid of the problem. An examination by you may determine the culprit, but a Veterinarian may be your only option for relief if the condition persists or seems debilitating.

PREVENTIVE MEASURES/CAUSES:
- Carefully check ears after hikes or running through bushes as foxtails, burrs or other matter could have gotten into the ears.
- Take care when cleaning ears that you don't squirt too much ear wash in that can't safely removed by you.
- When bathing dogs, insert large cotton balls to prevent water from entering the canal, and if your dog swims, do your best to dry out the inner ear afterwards -- even safely and gently clipping ears on top of head (if you can do so without hurting dog) for a ½ hour till the inside is nicely dried.
- Perform weekly exams of the ears so as to catch an infection early.

SIGNS & SYMPTOMS:
- Continuous head shaking, scratching or pawing at the ear
- Head tilt

WHAT YOU MAY NEED:
- Flashlight
- Ear wash
- Soft cloth or gauze

WHAT TO DO:
Take a good look inside. Upon inspection you may notice the ear looks dirty OR red and infected OR smells bad OR you may find tiny black specks that could be the dirt from ear mites. If it seems dirty or there is wax build-up, give it a thoroughly cleaning as described in the Head-to-Tail exam portion of this book on page 106 by pouring ear wash (or room temperature green or chamomile tea) onto a soft cloth and cleaning no deeper than the first knuckle on your index finger – no cotton swabs and take care not to push infection or debris into ear canal. If that doesn't do the trick, get to your Veterinarian for assistance. Middle ear infections can invade facial nerves and lead to facial paralysis; chronic infections can result in hearing loss and balance issues as well as meningitis, so don't delay in getting professional medical help.

If your pet has been outside there could also be foxtails or burrs trapped deep in the canal that only your Veterinarian can safely reach.

If you notice a Hematoma (where the ear flap fills with fluid creating a bubble-like swelling – like a giant blood blister), get your pet veterinary care as an infection or irritation deep down may have caused your dog to shake his head banging the ears against a wall or other surface. Your Veterinarian will treat the infection and hopefully aspirate the hematoma relieving both problems for your dog.

A head tilt may indicate a neurological problem, ear infection, irritation or be due to a toxin. Look inside your dog's ear and perform the tracking test learned on page 106, but most likely the best step is for your four-legged patient to receive medical care.

HEAT STROKE

Mary loved her Dachshund Daisy and always wanted her by her side. One 80°F day, the girls went for a car ride and Mary decided to stop at a convenience store for a jug of milk. Inside she encountered the cashier having difficulty at the register. The line of impatient customers grew, and Mary was delayed returning to her precious Doxie. Ten minutes passed. When Mary got out to the car, Daisy was panting profusely. Her gums were bright red, and she had little bits of foam around her mouth. Daisy was suffering from heat stroke!

CONDITION OVERVIEW:
It only takes a short period of time for an animal left in a car to get into a deadly situation. Dogs don't sweat to regulate their body temperature (normally 100.0°F − 102.5°F). They release heat through their tongue, nose and foot pads. Dogs pant to exchange cooler outside air with the warm humid air in their lungs while cats don't usually pant until they are overwhelmed by the heat. If the outside air isn't cooler than an animal's body temperature, the animal can succumb to heat stroke. Without prompt attention, heat stroke can result in brain damage, kidney failure, cardiac arrest and death.

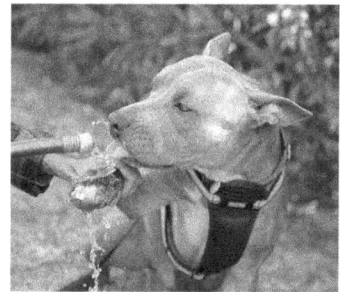
Photo by: Jackie Monell

Older and overweight dogs as well as short-nosed breeds are at the greatest risk.

PREVENTIVE MEASURES/CAUSES:
- Walk dogs during the cooler parts of the day and stick to shady areas and grass. Even beach sand can burn paws and make a canine body too hot!
- Always make sure pets have a supply of cool fresh water. If that outdoor water bowl has become a bird bath, is empty or is sitting in the blazing sun, it is not a good source of hydration for Fido!
- Make sure dogs in fenced yards always have shade to retreat to. Notice the situation at different times of the day and year to make sure the shade cast by your lovely backyard tree isn't only on the other side of the fence in the neighbor's yard leaving your dog in the hot sun.
- NEVER leave an animal in a parked car for even a moment. If he can't get out with you at every stop, he is better off home in a temperate environment.
- Remember heating systems in winter can make dogs too hot.
- Get to know your groomer! Blow drying dogs in a well-ventilated area is important to their health, and cage dryers (big boxes animals lie in with air forced in to dry them) must be carefully monitored, so choose a groomer you know has your pet's best interest at heart.
- Pay particular attention to senior, over-weight and brachycephalic (flat-faced) dogs who have more difficulty breathing even at comfortable temperatures.

SIGNS & SYMPTOMS:
- Heavy panting
- Gasping
- Vomiting (if not yet dehydrated)
- Foam around the mouth
- Weak or high pulse
- Inability to drink
- Bright red or suddenly bluish gums
- Loss of consciousness

Heat stroke is a life-threatening emergency that requires veterinary treatment. The goal is to remove the dog from the source of the heat, prevent internal body temperature from continuing to rise and transporting to a Veterinarian as quickly as possible.

WHAT YOU MAY NEED:
- Water from a garden hose, tub, wading pool, sink, even a spray bottle but make sure it's not hot from being in the sun
- Thermometer and lubricating gel
- Karo Syrup® or Honey

WHAT TO DO:
Move the dog to a cooler environment. Indoors is best with a cool fan blowing on your pet but even a shady sidewalk or grassy area can help.

Wet the animal with luke-warm water (not ice to avoid additional shock - see page 213). Think "From the paws up!" getting the paws, pits, groin and belly skin cooled first is most effective in bringing down the dog's body temperature. Water often skids off fur on breeds with undercoats and does not cool skin when applied to their back.

If you place your dog into a tub or pool, do not let the water rise higher than the belly. Immersing him to the neck will cause him to cool too quickly resulting in hypothermia.

Rubbing alcohol or witch hazel wiped onto the inner flaps of the ears and pads of the feet has an amazing cooling effect. Do not however douse a dog with an entire bottle of rubbing alcohol which could cause a sudden change in body temperature and result in shock. Also avoid getting in any cuts or scrapes as both sting.

Placing a cool pack (or bag of frozen peas) on the dog's neck and groin can prove helpful in cooling him off as the cooled blood flowing to major arteries cools the rest of the body. Remove pack every few minutes to make sure you don't cause frost bite to animal's tissue.

Do not force dogs to drink as he could aspirate fluid into his lungs. Dribble a little water from an eye dropper or spray bottle to keep him hydrated. At the Veterinarian's office, fluids will likely be administered subcutaneously (under the skin or intravenously).

Check your dog's temperature and if it is 104°F or higher, get to the Veterinarian immediately! Wrap the dog in wet sheet or towel, turn on car air conditioning and drive quickly but safely.

If the dog goes unconscious, rub a little honey or Karo Syrup® on his gums to increase blood sugar level, and be prepared to administer CPCR.

If the dog cools too quickly and temperature drops to 100°F, cover him with a blanket and place a 2-liter bottle filled with warm (not hot) water next to him as you transport him to the Animal ER.

HOMEOPATHIC TIP: *Belladonna*, a fever reducer also known as Night Shade, can prove beneficial in bringing temperature down but not as quickly as water and proper environment.

HOT SPOTS & LICK SORES

Summer sores, acute moist dermatitis, lick granulomas, acral lick dermatitis, OCLD (obsessive compulsive licking disorder). A hot spot by any name is still a painful nuisance to an animal in your care and often difficult to heal. Lick sores seem to appear spontaneously, and are generally found in easier-to-reach locations where a pet licks a small irritation and creates a flare up.

Veterinarians often cannot prescribe a specific cure since way down to the base layer of the skin, microscope pockets of bacteria and any combination of broken hair follicles, plugged and scarred oil glands and dilated and inflamed capillaries are present. If surgically removed, the pet then licks at the sutures or incision line creating a brand new granuloma, and the cycle repeats.

Hot spots occur when a dog itches, scratches and licks himself excessively forming a wet opening on the skin. Normal healthy bacteria are always present on an animal's body, but once he bites or chews and breaks the skin's surface, if there is even a little moisture, the perfect environment for bacterial contamination exists! Hot spots often form on the top of a dog's wrist joint or one of his paws – easy to lick spots – but can also be found on the hind legs and even ear flaps, especially in breeds with floppy ears. Affected pets generally have an allergic reaction, irritation or other underlying skin condition that starts them on an itch-lick-chew cycle. Some however, chew and lick purely out of boredom or as self-stimulation to alleviate separation anxiety. The pet becomes fixated and compulsively licks until a wound develops.

PREVENTIVE MEASURES/CAUSES:
- Lick sores occur more frequently during humid weather, after a bath or swim or when an animal walks in the rain, so it is imperative to keep pets clean and well-groomed.

- Pay attention to the smallest of sores, as even a slighting oozing wound can provide enough moisture for the bacteria to take hold.

- Irritation from matted fur can also cause these bothersome lesions to develop in any breed but particularly in those with dense undercoats.

- Parasite prevention is key as the itchiness caused by fleas and ticks leads to your dogs chewing himself raw.

- Does your dog have OCLD? Stop Obsessive Compulsive Licking Disorder in its tracks!

HOMEPATHIC TIP: Neem seed oil and human grade diatomaceous earth can keep fleas away from your dogs. Insect-borne diseases can be a serious health risk to people and pets but there is controversy over the safety of applying commercial insecticides so these can be effective alternatives.

SIGNS & SYMPTOMS:
- Compulsive licking and chewing at a particular body part
- Raised, rough, raw-looking lesion, typically on the top of a lower front leg or paw (but can be anywhere the pet can reach to lick or scratch)
- Reddish-brown saliva staining around the hot spot site
- Oozing, ulcerated, pus-filled drainage tracts coming from the hot spot site
- Foul smell coming from the hot spot site
- Swelling around the hot spot site
- Pain and visible discomfort

WHAT YOU MAY NEED:
- Scissors
- Gauze squares
- Green tea bag
- Warm water
- Antibacterial spray or cream
- Apple cider vinegar

WHAT TO DO:
1. Trim the fur around the hot spot with blunt nosed scissors. Exposing it to air will help dry out the moisture and speed healing.

2. Clean the area with a mild water-based astringent or antiseptic spray, even pure saline.

3. Gently pat the area dry with a soft cloth. Do not apply ointments to a hot spot as these products seal in infection while medications containing alcohol will burn an open wound. Instead use an antibacterial spray that dries up the sore or apply a tea bag (green, not herbal, that has cooled after being soaked for 5 minutes in hot water). The tannic acid is a natural astringent that dries and heals. Use this treatment 3-5 times per day until healed.

An alternate remedy is to apply apple cider vinegar (the unadulterated organic kind containing sediment) directly to the hot spot 4 times daily. Soak a cloth and wipe the clipped area gently. Apple cider vinegar has anti-inflammatory as well as antibacterial properties.

From your Pet First Aid Kit, apply hydrocortisone spray or cream (not ointment – see #3 above) to stop the itching and help promote healing.

4. Prevent pet from licking, chewing or scratching the affected area. Elizabethan or cervical collar might just be the tool needed. Although t-shirts, socks and doggie onesies help with some wounds, remember for hot spots, we want to keep them open to dry out.

5. Keep an eye on the area to make sure it continues to heal and doesn't worsen or spread. Hot spots often require a visit to the vet, who will likely prescribe topical medication usually in the form of a Gentamicin/Betamethasone spray and possibly oral antibiotics. It's possible the vet may also give the pet a cortisone injection to jump start the healing process.

IN HEAT (refer to "Birthing" section page 149 if you are passed this stage)

CONDITION OVERVIEW:
Estrus, or "heat" is the stage in a dog reproductive cycle during which she becomes receptive to mating. Her estrogen levels first increase and then sharply decrease, and mature eggs are released from the ovaries. The first "heat" usually occurs between 6 and 24 months of age and then occurs twice yearly in dogs. Each cycle lasts between 6-10 days, however, the female is only receptive to the male during the last half of this period. The male, however, may be interested the whole time.

PREVENTIVE MEASURES/CAUSES:
- Unless you are a responsible breeder willing to find forever homes for all the dogs born, spay your female (and neuter your males) before her first heat cycle to avoid possible health complications as well as to prevent the birth of more animals when so many already need homes.
- While "in heat," keep your female inaccessible to males realizing that if there is a male in the neighborhood, he will perform due diligence to get to your female.
- Know your breed. Any pregnant female should receive veterinary care, but breeds with larger heads (Boston Terriers & Pugs) often need C-sections to safely deliver their young as the wide heads could cause great trauma to their mom or prevent delivery altogether. If you allow your dog to become pregnant, it is your responsibility to see her and her puppies through it comfortably and with all medical care necessary.

SIGNS & SYMPTOMS:

- During estrus your female my act nervous, be easily distracted or even more alert than usual. She may feel the need to urinate more frequently and will exhibit changes in her behavior caused by the shift in hormones.
- Blood-tinged discharge may come from the vagina and the vulva will appear swollen.
- Discharge will decrease and lighten in color when she is ready to initiate sexual interactions with her suitors.
- Female may offer her hind-quarters towards approaching males.

WHAT YOU MAY NEED:

- Disinfectant and paper towels to clean up floors from any discharge
- Doggie diapers may help keep floors and carpets clean
- Good containment to keep male dogs away
- A calm & knowledgeable demeanor as well as other helping hands

WHAT TO DO:

Prevention is the key – spay your dog, but your most important task is to keep your female indoors and safe from escapes where she could be lost, injured or hit by a car while in search of a "boyfriend."

Offer diversions but spend time with your Miss. Keep doors and windows and fences secured.

Keep your female friend clean and mask the smell -- Chlorophyll tablets may help mask the odor of her cycle and keep Romeos away.

If dogs have mated, NEVER attempt to separate them. After the act, it is common for dogs to remain "connected" back-to-back for up to 30 minutes. You may endanger the dogs and/or be bitten if you interfere once nature has taken its course, so just allow them to remain safe and do not interfere until they separate on their own.

MANGE

CONDITION OVERVIEW:
Mange is an inflammatory condition caused by the Demodex Mite (various types so tiny you cannot seem them with the naked eye). Mange can cause a small, red, hairless area or almost complete hair loss (alopecia) with big pimples and thickened oozing skin. It can sometimes even disrupt the immune system. Mange occurs when mites burrow under the hair follicles and skin. Demodectic mange is much more common in dogs than in cats and typically causes hair loss and scaling around the eyelids, corners of the mouth and front legs. A second form called Canine Sarcoptic Mange or Scabies occurs when dogs are exposed to an infected animal at a kennel, dog park, shelter or wherever other dogs congregate. This type of mange is very contagious (to humans and animals) and very itchy. Only your Veterinarian can tell you for sure which type of mange your dog has, so see him right away and be patient in getting it resolved.

PREVENTIVE MEASURES/CAUSES:
- Keep your dogs well-groomed and parasite-free, and keep them more than paws reach away from any animal known to have mange.
- Don't breed dogs with chronic conditions of mange as it is likely to be passed on to offspring. .

SIGNS & SYMPTOMS:
- Redness
- Hair loss
- Pimples
- Crusty areas
- Itchiness/Scratching

WHAT YOU MAY NEED:
A trip to the vet! Only your Veterinarian can determine which type of mange your pet has and therefore the treatment necessary. Skin scrapings and maybe a few hairs will need to be looked at under the microscope. Blood and urine tests may be taken to determine underlying conditions.

WHAT TO DO:
Follow veterinary instructions…Special dips for your dog and his siblings may be in order. Launder bedding and keep your pooch clean and well fed (a healthy diet means a healthier animal – mange often affects dogs that are poorly nourished).

Fatty acid supplements (Omega 3s) are popular for skin disorders so discuss with your Veterinarian and often an antihistamine can help control the itch (1mg per pound of pet's body weight).

MOUTH SORES & ULCERS

CONDITION OVERVIEW:
Mouth sores can occur in older pets who have kidney or liver disease, diabetes or suffer from pancreatic tumors. They can become inflamed, be painful and prevent your pet from eating. Dental disease though too is often the culprit, but of course sores can occur anytime there is a cut, scrape or injury of any type to the mouth. Even allergies and mange around the mouth can result in sores, bumps and redness.

PREVENTIVE MEASURES/CAUSES:
- Examine your dog's mouth weekly so as to discover a small issue before it becomes a big painful problem.
- Brush your dog teeth at least 3 times a week to prevent gingivitis, abscesses and infections. Use a dog-specific tooth brush and dog-specific tooth paste as human toothpaste can be toxic to our four-legged friends.
- Schedule regular veterinary visits but also do not hesitate to seek medical advice at the first sign of symptoms.

SIGNS & SYMPTOMS:
- Excessive drooling or panting
- Not eating or difficulty chewing
- Bad breath
- Foaming at the mouth
- Frequent gagging
- Pawing at face
- Teeth grinding
- Bloody discharge from mouth or visible sores
- Crusty nose or bleeding from the nose

WHAT YOU MAY NEED:
- Saline or purified water to clean
- Soft warm-to-cool foods (baby food)
- Anbesol®
- Saline solution

WHAT TO DO:
To treat the problem, you need the advice of your Veterinarian, but you can help to relieve some pain for your precious friend by providing a topical treatment like Anbesol® and dabbing it directly on the sore. Crushed ice or ice water may also offer temporary relief, but watch your dog -- too hot or too cold foods or liquids may be painful. Providing softer meals will allow your dog to get his much-needed nutrition!

Follow your vet's prescribed treatment but notice any sign of infection. Rinsing your dog's mouth with saline solution may help speed up the healing process but don't wash away beneficial medication.

MUSCLE & JOINT INJURIES (Breaks, Sprains and Strains)

CONDITION OVERVIEW:
Since most dog parents do not have immediate access to an x-ray machine when their pet begins limping, you may not know if the animal has experienced a broken bone, muscle or tendon tear or strain. A broken bone (which requires emergency veterinary care) results when the bone cracks or actually separates due to trauma. A compound fracture (broken bone that has penetrated the skin) can cause severe bleeding and result in infection while sprains and strains occur when a ligament is over-stretched. Although painful, they often resolve on their own without surgical intervention. Should a ligament become torn, it will require surgical repair. All of these injuries are painful and can cause a great deal of swelling and distress to your dog.

PREVENTIVE MEASURES/CAUSES:
- Keep dogs fit and warm-up their muscles walking and stretching (refer to page 19 in this book) before they participate in rigorous running and jumping.
- Do your doggone best to avoid falls.
- Provide ramps in place of stairs especially for older pets, Dachshunds and Basset Hounds who are more prone to spinal disc injuries. This includes getting in and out of cars, on and off sofas, beds, anywhere they could place pressure or strain joints and muscles when jumping or climbing.
- Walk dogs on-leash or in fenced yards so they cannot escape and be hit by cars.
- Small pets tossed during animal fights can suffer bone and joint injuries so keep out of harm's way.

SIGNS & SYMPTOMS:
- Acute/sudden lameness or limping accompanied by pain
- Swelling at the joint
- Scrapes or wounds around the joint due to trauma to the area
- Heat, tenderness and/or swelling at the joint
- Bone protrusion

WHAT YOU MAY NEED:
- Sam splint® or other splinting materials (rolled magazine/newspaper, popsicle sticks, unsharpened pencils, wooden spoons, bubble wrap) depending on pet's size
- Flexible conforming wrap
- Gauze squares & rolls
- Antibacterial soap
- Water
- Antacid-coated aspirin (dogs only with Veterinarian's permission)
- Cold pack
- Board, towel or other means to transport pet
- Muzzle

WHAT TO DO:

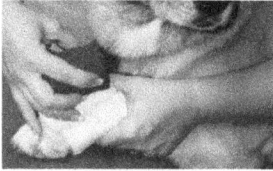

Photo by: Sunny-dog Ink

If small cuts or scrapes surround the joint, gently wash with antibacterial soap to clean and pat dry. If bleeding, apply direct pressure as discussed on page 140.

If pain level seems minimal and assumption is a slight strain, check with your Veterinarian about administering a mild pain reliever such as a coated aspirin for dogs only and make sure your dog is confined in a small room or crate to ensure rest. Apply a cold pack to any swelling four times daily for 5-10 minute
increments. Stop however if this is causing pain or distress. If not better the next day, PAWSitively see your Veterinarian.

If injury appears more serious or your dog is in considerable pain, lift him into car if he will stay calm, and get veterinary assistance. If however he is anxiously moving and may cause further injury to the joint or leg, splinting may be in order:

If you suspect a break (bone penetrating skin or a limb is hanging loosely), immobilize the limb immediately by securing a rolled-up newspaper to a large dog's leg or a popsicle stick to a small dog's limb with gauze and/or self-adhering wrap. Muzzling may be important to prevent a nip. Do not attempt to apply any kind of immobilization device if the animal is resistant or in extreme pain as you could do further damage or be bitten. Seek professional veterinary help immediately.

HOMEOPATHIC TIPS: For bruising, *Arnica Montana* (Leopard's bane) is an alternative choice. It can be applied as a salve or cream or dosed as a tincture – 30c - 200c every four to twelve hours is the general starting point. Stop when you see improvement, but if there is no improvement in a few days, stop as well and obtain professional medical care.

NOSEBLEEDS

CONDITION OVERVIEW:
Known as epistaxis in the medical world, nosebleeds may come on suddenly (acute) or be longer-term in nature (chronic); they may affect one or both nostrils but usually are the result of trauma due to the sensitive nasal cavities common in our dogs.

Sometimes nosebleeds are caused by a condition known as coagulopathy, where blood just does not clot as it should. Other possibilities include wounds, an internal injury which is not visible, a tumor, cancer in an organ or Leukemia. Ingesting rat poison, injury due to a foreign object or Canine Erlichiosis (bacterial disease contracted from ticks) as well as Rocky Mountain Spotted Fever (also from ticks) may cause nosebleeds to occur. If you see blood coming from your pet's nostrils, a prompt visit to your Veterinarian is a must.

PREVENTIVE MEASURES/CAUSES:
- Keep dogs away from sharp and poisonous objects.
- Keep your dogs tick-free.
- Do weekly head-to-tail check-ups of your pet to find problems when they are small.
- Always give your dog the once over after a hike to make sure foxtails, burrs or even pieces of grass aren't stuck in nose, ears or other body parts.

SIGNS & SYMPTOMS:
- Bloody discharge from the nostrils
- Sneezing fits
- Difficulty breathing; wheezing
- Bad breath which could indicate a dental problem may be the cause

WHAT YOU MAY NEED:
- Cold compress
- Gauze squares

WHAT TO DO:
As for any injury or illness, keep your dog calm! Heavy panting or excited sneezing may exacerbate the bleeding.

Apply a cold compress and apply direct pressure with an absorbent cloth.

Never use a muzzle during a nosebleed but do try to keep dog as calm as possible so that he doesn't shake his head.

Call your Veterinarian and take your dog in if advised. Medication or even cauterization of the blood vessels may be in order as well as testing for the exact cause.

OBESITY/OVERWEIGHT

CONDITION OVERVIEW:

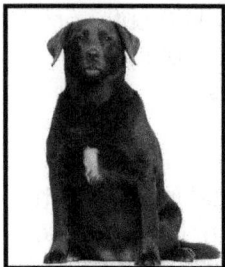

The Association for Pet Obesity Prevention has determined that more than half of our dogs are overweight. Additionally, research shows a correlation between overweight pets and overweight owners. Fitness is important on two-legs and four-paws! Generally, lack of exercise combined with overeating is the main culprit, but there can by underlying health conditions, so start off by taking your plump pooch or extra fluffy feline to the Veterinarian for a check-up to make sure all systems are go for an exercise program. Even a few extra pounds increase the risk of heart disease, diabetes, respiratory illness and joint problems in your four-legged best friend as in yourself, so start slowly, but grab a leash, slip on your walking shoes and get those paws and legs moving for a healthy lifetime together.

PREVENTIVE MEASURES/CAUSES:

- Know WHAT you are putting into your dog's body. Read pet food labels (see page 14) looking for a high quality protein as the first ingredient (unless prescribed otherwise by your Veterinarian) and low to no carbohydrates. Learn which human foods are good and which are not for your pet and get better educated on canine nutrition remembering EVERY body is different and all of your dogs, even if from the same litter, may not thrive on the same food. Allergies, differing metabolisms and other conditions may require every dog in the household to have a diet especially tailored to them.
- Hup two three four, hup two three…all you doggies walk with me! Get those paws moving but start off slowly realizing pets too need to be conditioned and work up to a more rigorous routine. Pay attention to your pets, not pushing too hard. Several 10-20 minute walks daily are better than a one hour long one, especially if you have seniors.
- Don't miss annual check-ups at your Veterinarian. Blood tests and urinalysis may determine kidney, thyroid and other problems early and help you find a solution.

SIGNS & SYMPTOMS:

Your dog may be overweight if:
- you can't feel his ribs easily under his fur coat (you shouldn't however be able to see ribs on most breeds).
- his belly hangs lower than his chest
- he doesn't have a waistline when you look down at his back from your eye level
- he has become a couch potato or tires quickly with minimal exercise

Don't use the excuse that he's not fat, just fluffy -- you are doing your dog a disservice and may be shortening his life!

WHAT YOU MAY NEED:

- There is no magic pill or quick fix! Experts will lead you on the path, so depending on the suggested course of action, you may need a new diet, new collar and leash, exercise equipment, water therapy, etc.

- Low calorie treats -- slices of raw zucchini, apples, carrots and broccoli -- are smarter choices than fat-filled flour based biscuits.

WHAT TO DO:
First, get a good check-up at the Veterinarian for the go-ahead to begin a better exercise program. Also discuss diet and contact a canine nutritionist for the best tips and advice.

Check into the unlimited resources at your disposal but start at a speed comfortable for your pet. You too may tone up and drop a pound or two thanks to your work-out partner!

POISONING

CONDITION OVERVIEW:
Dogs love to chew. That spray bottle, aerosol can or other container under your cabinet can be deadly if an animal punctures it and ingests the liquid inside. Knowing what to do and having the necessary tools on hand can avert a minor injury or a major disaster.

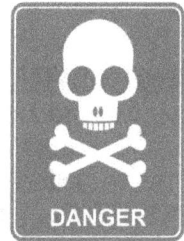

Size does matter when it comes to poisoning. What could kill a Chihuahua may have no effect on a Saint Bernard. The ability for any potentially poisonous substance to cause health issues is proportional to the animal's body weight. Additionally, every item on a poison list may not harm every animal, but, if it has made the list, a significant number of animals have had an adverse reaction to it, so err on the side of caution for your dog's sake.

Chocolate accounts for 50% of the calls received by the Pet Poison Helpline. It is most poisonous to dogs, cats and ferrets. Although antioxidants in dark chocolate are considered good for human hearts, the darker the chocolate, the worse it is for many animals. The culprit is theobromine -- both a cardiac stimulant and a diuretic, which can speed up the heart while pulling fluids from the body resulting in rapid heart rate and breathing, vomiting, diarrhea, seizures and even death.

One ounce of milk chocolate per pound of body weight can be fatal to dogs. The darker the chocolate, the higher the concentration of theobromine which means the less it takes to have the same ill effects.

The basic formula is below, but realize some dogs are more sensitive and can be harmed by less than the amount provided on a chart:
- Milk Chocolate – 1 ounce per pound of body weight
- Dark Chocolate – ½ ounce per pound of body weight
- Baker's (unsweetened) Chocolate – ¼ ounce per pound of body weight
- Dry Cocoa Powder – 1/8 ounce (less than one teaspoon) per pound of body weight
- Cocoa Bean Mulch – Due to the variation in manufacturing, the concentration of theobromine can vary depending on the manufacturer. However, if you suspect that a dog in your care has ingested cocoa bean mulch, seek veterinary advice.

PREVENTIVE MEASURES/CAUSES:

- Every year thousands of pets needlessly suffer, and many die, from ingesting substances in our homes and even from human food. Be proactive in making sure that an animal's environment is free of potentially hazardous substances:
  - Get down on all fours and look at life from your dog's point-of-view, (indoors and out), and keep harmful items out of paw's reach.
  - Install childproof locks on cabinet doors if you share your life with curious dogs.
  - Read labels and purchase "pet friendly" chemicals and cleaners.
  - Remember that when you have a dog, you have a four-legged toddler for life.

It is your responsibility to keep your dog safe and supervise where your dog goes and what they can get into.

SIGNS & SYMPTOMS:

- Vitals not normal (see page 103)
- Rapid or decreased heart rate
- Difficulty breathing or heavy panting (which also often indicates pain)
- Slow CRT -- Shock
- Muscle tremors or seizures
- Vomiting and/or diarrhea, sometimes with blood
- Drooling or foaming
- Pawing at the mouth
- Redness of the skin, ears, eyes, any body part
- Lethargy or anxiety
- Blisters or sores on the mouth or skin where poison made contact
- Swelling
- Elevated or decreased heart rate, breathing or body temperature
- Anything that is not normal for your pet!

WHAT YOU MAY NEED:

- Phone numbers for your Veterinarian and poison control easily accessible
- ASPCA Poison Control Center Hotline (888) 426-4435
- Pet Poison Helpline/VP (800) 213-6680 ... Fees Apply
- Know the weight of the animals in your care so that you can properly administer solutions (only on the advice of a Veterinarian).
- Needle-less Syringe, eye dropper or turkey baster
- Water or non-fat yogurt for diluting poison
- 3% Hydrogen peroxide for inducing vomiting
- Plastic zip lock bag to collect vomit sample

WHAT TO DO:

1. GATHER INFORMATION if you know (or suspect) that a pet has been poisoned:
   - Determine the type of poison, how much ingested and how long ago.
   - Check the animal's vital signs (temperature, heart rate, respiration, capillary refill time, gum color).

- Observe symptoms (difficulty breathing, vomiting, diarrhea, seizures, bleeding, etc).
- Stay calm and react to the situation in a reasonable manner. If possible, read the container label of the substance that you suspect the animal has ingested.
- Immediately call your Veterinarian or poison control and do exactly as instructed.

2. REACT – Induce vomiting or dilute poison in your pet's body
To induce vomiting (may be recommended if the animal has ingested food or non-caustic toxins – ones that don't burn):
- With your veterinarian's okay, give your dog fresh, bubbly, non-expired 3% Hydrogen Peroxide. It may however, irritate his stomach for up to two weeks after. Dosage is ½ - 1 teaspoon per 5 lbs. of the dog's body weight (1-2ml/kg). Also, 1 Tablespoon per 15 lbs. if that is an easier calculation.
- Once the dog has swallowed all of the hydrogen peroxide, have the dog stand in front of you and give him a vigorous belly-rub. He should vomit within 5 minutes. If not, you may administer a second dose, but if he does not vomit in 5-10 additional minutes, proceed quickly to veterinary help.
- If your dog vomits, collect a sample and take it, the poison container and your dog to the Veterinarian ASAP to be sure all toxins have left the body and that your pet is suffering no ill effects.

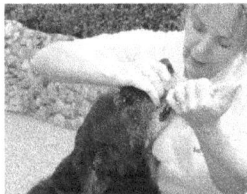

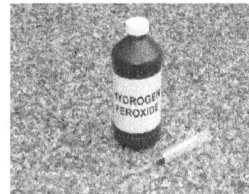

Photos by: Sunny-dog Ink

NOTE: *Do NOT use Salt, Syrup of Ipecac (can result in cardiac issues and prolonged vomiting), digital stimulation (fingers in the throat can cause injury to the animal), liquid dish soap, raw eggs, tabasco or any other creative techniques! Additionally, never administer activated charcoal (a binding agent) unless specifically told to do so by your Veterinarian. If the toxin ingested ends in the letters "ol" (such as xylitol, alcohol, glycol, etc.), the charcoal will not bind to it and achieve the desired effect. Emesis works best if performed within 2 hours of ingestion. Up to 50% of stomach contents may be evacuated. It's possible to induce vomiting later than that for grapes and raisins as they don't break down quickly, chocolate (which isn't readily absorbed), xylitol gum and bezoars (fur balls).*

Emesis is typically done for food items, medications, ingestions of large quantities, certain rodenticides and small dull objects in dogs, but as mentioned above, get dogs quickly to the veterinarian to have this procedure done with prescription-only medications.

CAUTION: *Do not induce vomiting in canines that have a history of aspiration, have congestive heart issues, are laterally recumbent or very lethargic as the potential for aspiration into the lungs is higher. Also be very careful with brachycephalic breeds for this same reason.*

*Final note: **Never induce vomiting if the dog has swallowed a sharp object, corrosive object (batteries) or hydrocarbons (gas, motor oil, kerosene)!***

To Dilute
If you suspect that the dog has ingested a potentially caustic substance, or if you have no idea what he may have swallowed, do not induce vomiting. Proceed immediately to your Veterinarian while getting fluids into your dog's body to dilute the toxic substance. Water or non-fat yogurt are generally the best options as many pets will vomit up cow's milk.

Other ways an animal can be poisoned:
In addition to what goes in their mouths, dogs can be poisoned by toxins that are absorbed, inhaled or injected into their bodies. Therefore, knowing what, where (which body part) and how much Fido got into determines your course of action.

- **Absorbed poisons** are substances that get on our dog's paws and coat and are absorbed through their skin. These poisons may also be ingested once the animal licks and grooms himself.
    - Wash the area thoroughly and visit your Veterinarian to prevent long-term effects and discomfort.
    - For oil-based toxins (petroleum products), use a gentle dishwashing liquid or shampoo before flushing with water.
    - If the poison is a dry powdery substance (such as sink scrubs or granulated swimming pool chlorine), brush or vacuum away before washing the area -- if you add water to a dry toxin, you will activate it ON your dog's skin! If the irritant is in your dog's eye, carefully flush the eye with purified water/eye wash.
- **Inhaled poisons** include aerosol sprays, carbon monoxide, gases, and other fumes inhaled into your dog's lungs. Quickly get the dog into fresh air and administer rescue breathing if needed by holding his mouth shut and breathing into his nostrils – every 2-3 seconds for animals 40 lbs and higher, while twice as quickly for smaller dogs giving tiny puff breaths.

- **Injected poisons** include insect stings and snake bites discussed in this book on pages 145-151.

Marijuana or cannabis poisoning, (not be confused with non-psychoactive CBD Oil), is on the rise with our dogs with a 30% increase in calls to the Animal Poison Control Center since 2009. It does not agree with dogs and although they may become sedated and act drunk like humans, many become agitated, have increased heart rates and are in major distress. They stagger around dribbling urine and may go into a coma and die without veterinary treatment. Keep in mind that marijuana butter, brownies and cookies can be doubly dangerous with their additions of fats and chocolates. Please keep all drugs, prescribed or non-prescribed, out of paw's reach!

For a list of Common Household Poisons, see page 235

PROLAPSE

CONDITION OVERVIEW:
A prolapse occurs when a part of the body (typically an internal structure) slips or moves out of place generally due to trauma or illness.

PREVENTIVE MEASURES/CAUSES:
Prevent fleas, worms and other parasites from invading your dogs as they could be the underlying cause of a prolapse.
Provide plenty of fresh clean water at all times to keep your dogs regular and ward off urinary infections.

Areas likely to prolapse are:
- Rectum – generally caused by straining/constipation or anaphylactic shock; rectal tumors and gastrointestinal parasites may also cause this form of prolapse.
- Urethra – usually occurs in young male dogs who have poorly developed urinary tracts.
- Penis – inability to completely retract into the sheath (aka paraphimosis).
- Vagina (may include the uterus) – generally due to straining associated with birth (whelping in dogs and queening in cats) or vaginal hyperplasia (swelling of tissue causing protrusion through the vulva); spaying can prevent vaginal prolapse.
- Eyes – often caused from too much pressure placed above the eye socket, especially in dogs with prominent eyes like Pugs or Pekingese.

SIGNS & SYMPTOMS:
- Protrusion of any body part from its normal location
- Dog may be licking or chewing at protrusion
- Pain/discomfort

WHAT YOU MAY NEED:
- K-Y® or other water soluble jelly
- Gauze
- Saline solution

WHAT TO DO:
Should you notice a protrusion, get your injured dog to prompt veterinary care. Do not try to push the protrusion back into place! The underlying cause must be determined by your Veterinarian who has the skill to then gently massage or surgically reposition the body part. Before you head out, soak gauze squares with saline solution and apply to the protruding area. This helps keep the organ's tissues from drying out and increases the chance that the Veterinarian will be able to revitalize the damaged organ tissue. Covering the body part also prevents the dog from chewing on the exposed area as does applying a cone collar to your furry patient.

When it is an eyeball that is displaced, the eyelid is curled back preventing the lid from covering the eye. Until you reach veterinary care, rinse the eye with saline every 5 minutes to prevent it from drying out.

For rectal or vaginal prolapse, you may apply water-soluble lubricating jelly to ease discomfort, but only let your Veterinarian attempt to reposition the prolapse.

In cases of paraphimosis, rinse the extruded penis with copious amounts of saline solution to help decrease inflammation of the tissues, then apply water-soluble lubricating jelly to the end. Gently moving any hairs that might be preventing retraction may allow it to return to its sheath. Medical intervention however is advised as the prepuce may constrict blood flow which could cause tissue death in the penis.

PUNCTURES & BITE WOUNDS

CONDITION OVERVIEW:

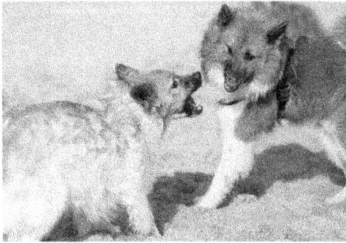

When objects pierce the skin (nails, teeth of another animal, glass, sharp sticks for instance), they leave small holes through which bacteria enters the body. Bite wounds are often disguised by fur and can develop into an abscess if they are not discovered and immediately treated. X-rays or ultrasounds might be needed to diagnose internal bleeding and damage, especially in the case of animal bites since the tearing of deep layers of muscle may have occurred. Large dogs are capable of inflicting bone crushing injuries. Deep injuries around the neck and chest are commonly seen if a smaller animal is picked up and shaken by a larger one.

De-gloving injuries result when skin is torn away and include significant tissue damage and blood loss. Dog suffer this injury from animal attacks, entanglement in barbed wire fencing and even being hit by cars. If blood supply is not quickly returned to the skin, necrosis (tissue death) may occur and skin grafting may become necessary.

PREVENTIVE MEASURES/CAUSES:
- Keep your home and yard free of sharp and dangerous debris, and keep your dog out of harm's way when using garden tools, saws, grass trimmers or any machinery.
- When walking your dog, keep your dog on-leash and keep your eyes peeled to the path ahead checking for glass and other sharp objects. Keeping him on-leash will also help keep him safe from injuries sustained by automobiles and other animals.
- Don't just sweep up broken glass…vacuum it too! Tiny shards could remain and pierce dog paws.

SIGNS & SYMPTOMS:
- Bleeding
- Skin cut, scraped or torn away
- Puncture
- Pain
- Limping
- Licking at body parts

WHAT YOU MAY NEED:

- 4 X 4 Gauze squares
- Gauze roll
- Self-adhering compression bandage or adhesive tape
- Saline solution
- Antibacterial Soap, Chlorhexidine, Hibiclens®

WHAT TO DO:

Stop bleeding by applying direct pressure. If the wound is not bleeding, rinse with saline solution or antibacterial soap. Puncture wounds that penetrate all layers of the skin can allow bacteria to penetrate deeply into the body. As the tissue begins to close, the bacteria can quickly get trapped and cause infection, so get to your Veterinarian.

If the puncture is from an animal bite, find out if other animal is current on his vaccinations (if possible). Pain, redness and infection can occur around untreated areas and your dog may develop a fever, loss of appetite and become lethargic. Antibiotics most likely will be needed to get him through this episode.

Punctures to the Chest (Sucking Chest Wounds)

CONDITION OVERVIEW:

The cavity inside your dog's chest normally allows the lungs to easily expand when air is inhaled. However, when an object protrudes the chest wall, air gets sucked into the chest cavity and that pressure collapses the lungs, preventing them from expanding and resulting in suffocation. This sort of injury, caused by a bite or piercing object (including a knife, bullet, arrow, stick or even a broken rib), is commonly called a sucking wound because of the way air is pulled into the hole made by the object. Even if nothing appears to have punctured a dog's chest, if you hear a gurgling sound and/or see frothy blood, something (most likely a rib) has penetrated. *You have a life-threatening emergency to help your pet through. You must get veterinary help but following the "What To Do" steps below can help...*

PREVENTIVE MEASURES/CAUSES:

- Do your doggone best to keep dogs out of harm's way...NEVER allow them where hunting or even recreational sporting events take place. Bullets, arrows and even BB guns can fatally wound or seriously injure your dog.
- Keep dogs safe when working with yard equipment. Rocks and other debris can fly out of lawnmowers and grass trimmers causing puncture injuries.
- Only allow your dog around other animals you know and watch out for wildlife. Don't let pets roam freely, especially at nighttime. It only takes seconds for the worst to happen.
- If a dog has been hit by a car or struck in the chest, assume he could have a sucking wound to the chest (possibly due to a broken rib penetrating the lung), so quickly and carefully assess and get professional help.

SIGNS & SYMPTOMS:
- Bubbling of blood at chest site
- Slow breathing or fast and labored
- Abdomen may move more with each breath
- Dog may try stretching neck to facilitate breathing

WHAT YOU MAY NEED:
- Gauze squares
- Gauze rolls
- K-Y Jelly® or other water soluble gel
- Honey or Karo® syrup
- Plastic wrap
- Adhesive tape or self-adhering wrap
- Towels/blankets

WHAT TO DO:
Your goal is to make a one-way valve that prevents air from being sucked into the chest cavity. You want to re-establish the normal "vacuum" that should exist in the cavity, prevent lung collapse and help pet breathe easy until medical help is available.

1) Treat your pet for shock (see page 213) after checking CRT (page 105). Keep him warm and put a drop or two of honey or Karo® Syrup on his gums.

2) If the wound has a small opening, seal it with a big glob of K-Y Jelly® to prevent incoming air from collapsing the lung.

3) Place clean gauze or plastic wrap (even a plastic baggie will suffice) on top of the opening and hold in place with tape on 3 of the 4 sides. When the dog inhales, his lungs will push air out of the chest cavity and back through the hole, so your bandaging will need to lift on that one side to release air from the body. When the dog exhales, and the lungs deflate, the sucking wound will pull the plastic back against the hole and prevent additional air from entering the chest and collapsing the lung.

4) If the wound is too large for water soluble lubricating jelly, cover tightly with plastic wrap to form a seal and tape it in place. If possible, have the pet lie on the injured side to keep pressure on the bleeding and help seal the hole.

5) *Get Immediate Veterinary Attention.*

REVERSE SNEEZE

CONDITION OVERVIEW:
Known as Inspiratory Paroxysmal Respiration or Pharyngeal Gag Reflex, a reverse sneeze comes on suddenly and causes the dog to extend his head and neck while making rapid inspiratory movements (inhalations), generally with his mouth closed causing "snorting" sounds to come from the nasal passages. Often referred to as a backward sneeze in which irritation causes the soft palate to spasm, it may be due to irritation in the sinuses but most often remains a mystery, even to the most competent Veterinarians. Although it sounds distressing to pet parents, it is generally not harmful and most dogs appear completely normal before and after an episode. Reverse sneezing commonly occurs during or following a nap, exercise or meals, although for many dogs, there is just no pattern. Most episodes are truly random but could be caused by chemical irritants, nasal mites, post-nasal drip or even a blade of grass or other material stuck back in the nasal area (retropharynx). Although it can sound similar to the honking noise a pet makes due to a collapsed trachea, reverse sneezes generally subside quickly on their own.

PREVENTIVE MEASURES/CAUSES:
- None really but provide a dust-free environment for any pet prone to this ailment.
- Have your Veterinarian check-out your dog to rule out certain underlying causes.

SIGNS & SYMPTOMS:
- Rapid and long inspirations (inhaling) resulting in a loud snorting sound.
- Dog stands still and may extend his head and/or neck forward as the trachea may have narrowed during the spasm and he is trying to get more air.

WHAT YOU MAY NEED:
- Patience. Episodes generally subside in a matter of minutes, but stand by in case this is only the beginning to a bigger problem.

WHAT TO DO:
Encourage your pet to drink water, but do not force him to.

Gently massage the throat in a downward motion and/or momentarily cover the nostrils or blow a puff of air into the dog's face as all these methods make the dog swallow allowing him to clear the irritation and relax the spasm.

Most dogs just need the spasm to run its course of 20-30 seconds to several minutes.

Once the sneezing stops, most pets return to normal with no ill effects. If yours does not however, seek veterinary care after immediately checking vitals (including capillary refill time) and making sure he is breathing. It's often a good idea to video an episode to show your Veterinarian for confirmation as you'll never get your dog to have a reverse sneeze on command in the doctor's office!

SECONDHAND SMOKE

CONDITION OVERVIEW/PRECAUTIONS:

Tobacco smoke exhaled by humans plus the actual smoke released from a pipe, burning cigarette or cigar contains thousands of chemicals including harmful ones like carbon monoxide, arsenic, formaldehyde and benzene. The last several decades have proven that people who are repeatedly exposed to environmental tobacco smoke are more likely to develop lung cancer, breathing and heart problems than those who are not exposed to these chemicals. Recent studies show similar findings in our companion dogs citing increased eye irritation, lung and nasal cancers in dogs who cohabitate with human smokers and who are subject to chronic exposure. Breeds with long noses (Collies and Afghans for instance) are at greater risk for nasal disease while our shorter snouted friends (Shih-Tzus, Bulldogs and Pugs) are more at risk for lung problems.

PREVENTIVE MEASURES/CAUSES:

- Make sure your dog has a clean sleeping and living environment. If you smoke, do so outside where it can dissipate and not linger where you dog lives and breathes.
- Make sure cigar and cigarettes and their discarded butts are kept out of paw's reach.
- An air purifier may help rid your home of harmful impurities for you and your dog, smoke or not. Antioxidants, such as vitamin C, can rid the body of some free-radicals.

SIGNS & SYMPTOMS:

- Red, irritated eyes (may paw at them)
- Raspy breaths; difficulty breathing
- Coughing, gasping sounds
- Coughing up blood or blood coming from nasal passages

WHAT YOU MAY NEED:

- Veterinary check-up!

WHAT TO DO:

Get to the Veterinarian and follow recommended treatment.

SEIZURES & CONVULSIONS

CONDITION OVERVIEW:
A seizure or convulsion is a sudden uncontrolled electrical activity in the brain that results in a series of involuntary muscle contractions and abnormal behaviors lasting from seconds to minutes. Severity can range from a glazed-over look in the eyes to twitching in a part of the face to the animal falling on his side, barking, gnashing his teeth, urinating, defecating and running in place while lying down. Seizures are symptoms of poisoning or a neurological disorder and are not in themselves a disease. The former "grand mal" and "petit mal" classifications have been replaced with "tonic" (stiffening & possible collapse) and "clonic" (actual convulsions). Psychomotor seizures manifest as unusual behaviors (ie: fly biting at air, staring into space) and are sometimes referred to as "absence spells" as the dog appears unaware of his surroundings.

PREVENTIVE MEASURES/CAUSES:
- Some seizures are idiopathic meaning the cause cannot be determined, but others are results of:
- Poisoning (chocolate, xylitol or or snail/slug bait pellets for instance)
- Low blood sugar
- Brain tumor or head trauma
- Liver disease
- Inflammation or an infectious disease of the nervous system
- Epilepsy (when all else is ruled out, this is the general diagnosis)
- Stress or extreme anxiety
- Distemper or Rabies

SIGNS & SYMPTOMS:
The 3 Stages of a Seizure
- **Aura** is the first stage and may occur seconds before to several days prior to a seizure. Restlessness, whining/crying, shaking, salivation, wandering aimlessly, hiding or even overly needy or affectionate signs may by demonstrated by your pet.
- **Ictus** is when the seizure occurs. You may notice a glazing over of the eyes and staring just as it is about to occur. We refer to this as "the lights are on, but nobody is home" look, which may last for seconds or hours.
- **Postictal** is the stage immediately following the seizure when the animal appears confused, disoriented and may be unresponsive. Dog may not have great control of motor skills or bodily functions and may need assistance getting up or walking and may stumble or easily fall.

WHAT YOU MAY NEED:
- Stop watch to time seizure
- A calm demeanor as your emotional state, and that of those around you, may affect the patient
- Towel to use as a sling to assist walking afterwards on large animals
- Baby gate (if this is an ongoing situation for your dog, you'll want to make sure he can't tumble down stairs)

WHAT TO DO:

Once a seizure starts, there is nothing you can do to stop it. The goal is to keep the dog from injuring itself.

- If other animals are in the vicinity, get them behind a closed door away from the seizing dog. Many animals, even the gentlest and most obedient, will attack a seizing animal as the seizure appears to them to be an act of aggression.
- Stay away from dog's mouth. During a seizure the dog will not be in voluntary control of its actions. However, the jaws perform involuntary muscle contractions, and if you get in the way, teeth will meet flesh.
- *Think CALM & COMFORTABLE or SOFT & SERENE*, whichever terms resonate with you.

  Toss SOFT/COMFORTABLE blankets or pillows around the dog for cushioning, especially if the seizure is happening on a hard surface; remove tables and chairs from next to the dog.

  Stay CALM and create a SERENE environment by reducing noise, anxiety and stimulation of any type (turn off televisions and stereo components, dim lights, close draperies over bright windows and remove angst-filled humans, and other animals from the area).

- Time the seizure (all three stages if possible). If this is a first-time seizure or unusually long for your epileptic dog, have him checked out by your Veterinarian. If multiple seizures are occurring in a 24-hour period, also get immediate veterinary help. If the seizure doesn't subside after a few minutes, the dog's body temperature can start to rise due to repeated muscle contractions. Heatstroke and hypoxia (low oxygen to the brain) are life-threatening. IV meds may be needed to stop the convulsions, so transport with great care, but get quickly to veterinary help.

Never leave a dog that has just experienced a seizure alone. If you have a dog prone to seizures that is home alone during parts of the day, make sure he stays in a safe room… free of sharp/hard corners and places he could get trapped in or fall from if disoriented. Install baby gates near stairways or even where there are only a few steps to prevent injuries.

SHOCK

CONDITION OVERVIEW:
Shock is a life-threatening condition that occurs when your dog does not get sufficient blood flow and oxygen to his tissues and organs. The body tries to compensate by increasing the heart and respiratory rates, restricting urinary output to maintain fluids and constricting blood vessels near the skin. All this requires additional energy the animal doesn't have since his vitals are not functioning properly and will result in death without quick medical care. Hypovolemic shock is when severe blood and fluid loss render the heart unable to pump sufficient blood to the body. Neurogenic shock, caused by a relaxation of muscles, causes blood pressure to drop and is usually the result of a severe spinal injury or electrocution.

PREVENTIVE MEASURES/CAUSES:
Know your dog! Causes of shock may include heart failure, sepsis (blood infection), anaphylactic shock, traumatic injury, dehydration and blood loss. When your pet does not appear right, immediately look at his gum color and check CRT (page 105) to determine if treatment for Shock is a priority!

SIGNS & SYMPTOMS:
- Capillary Refill Time exceeds 2 seconds (see page 105)
- Dog appears woozy or weak; as if over-exerted
- Panting
- Rapid heart rate
- Bright red gums

Late stage signs of shock include:
- Pale skin and gums – slow CRT (Capillary Refill Time)
- Drop in body temperature – cold extremities
- Slow respiratory rate
- Weak or absent pulse
- Depression or apathy
- Unconsciousness

WHAT YOU MAY NEED:
- Towel or blanket
- Honey or Karo Syrup®
- Electrolyte Solution (1/2 tsp salt, ½ tsp baking soda, 2 cups water)
- Immediate transport to Veterinarian

WHAT TO DO:
- Check capillary refill time (CRT) by pressing on the dog's gums. If it takes more than two seconds for pink color to return to gums (or if the gums are too pale to evaluate CRT), the dog may be experiencing shock.
- Elevate dog's hind quarters slightly by placing a pillow or folded blanket underneath to increase circulation. Do not elevate if you suspect a broken back or if there is a bleeding head or chest injury. In that case, lie flat or elevate area of wound if bleeding is heavy.

- Retain dog's body heat by covering him with a sheet or blanket, including a blanket underneath if surface beneath him is cold such as a tile floor, concrete or even the ground.
- Gently rub dog's gums with honey or Karo Syrup® to get glucose to the brain.
- Transport to a veterinary hospital immediately. Always call ahead to be assured they can accommodate you and that they are ready to help. Check ahead to see if you should administer electrolytes on the way (1/2 tsp per 30 lbs. of body weight every 30 minutes).

SKIN ALLERGIES & INFECTIONS

CONDITION OVERVIEW:
The skin is the body's first line of defense. It protects your dog from the outside elements including micro-organisms, prevents moisture loss and keeps his body thermo-regulated. Slightly thinner than our human skin, your pet's skin covers the blood and lymphatic vessels, nerves, sweat and sebaceous glands and hair follicles and is considered the largest organ of his body. It therefore goes through wear and tear and is subjected to bacteria, fungi and parasites as well as cuts and abrasions. Hormonal imbalances too can result in skin changes. Dogs can suffer from red, itchy, oily or flaky skin with or without hair loss to the area. Although medical treatment is often necessary to cure the problem, a great first step can be making your pet more comfortable. Scratching and chewing are amongst the biggest summertime complaints dog owners share with their Veterinarians. Skin allergies (which can lead to infections) are generally caused by either fleas (or other parasites/insects), food or environment (grass, pollens, chemicals on floors, bedding or lawns). They result in non-stop itching, scratching and then open sores that take forever to heal. Masking the itch may help your pet find relief, but getting to the underlying cause is the only way to break this vicious and uncomfortable cycle.

PREVENTIVE MEASURES/CAUSES:
Bathe your dog frequently. Confer with your Veterinarian and Groomer to determine how often: 1-2 times per month may be necessary to remove yeast and keep your dog's skin clean. A good brushing several times per week can help remove dirt and distribute oils evenly throughout your pet's skin and coat.

Perform a weekly Head-to-Tail check-up (page 49) so that you can more readily find a small scrape, a burr or foxtail or any sign of problem on your best friend.

Use monthly parasite preventives to keep fleas, ticks and the resulting allergies and bacteria at bay. Even if you don't see fleas, it doesn't mean they are not biting your four-legged friend. Get out a flea comb (tiny close together tines or teeth) and brush at the base of your dog's tail. If you get tiny dark specks, place them on a damp paper towel and if it turns pink... those specs are, in fact, flea dirt containing the dried blood of your pet! Some dogs can develop an allergy after only a few bites, so use the monthly flea preventive your Veterinarian recommends and use it according to instructions -- dog's body weight, species (never dog meds on cats for instance) and frequency.

Other dogs develop hypersensitivities to components in their diets. Wheat, corn, beef and chicken can turn some dogs into scratching fools. Canine nutritionists (experts trained beyond the level of most Veterinarians in regards to a pet's diet) are recommending novel (new) proteins such as lamb, venison and ostrich. A diagnosis requires food trials so you may need to start eliminating an ingredient every few weeks from your dog's diet to determine what is causing the negative reaction. If the itching subsides, you have determined the ingredient that doesn't work with Fido's system. You can slowly add some of those ingredients back in, one at a time, and if the itching reoccurs, you've determined the culprit!

As for the environment, grass, weeds, pollen, mold spores, dust mites, fertilizers, insecticides, carpet powder and laundry detergent can irritate your dog and make him scratch his paws off. Intradermal tests can be performed at your Veterinarian's office. Although cortisone and/or steroid injections may ease the itch, knowing what is causing it and keeping it away from your pet is the best solution. A good old-fashioned oatmeal bath and calamine lotion may help him find relief in the meantime, and adding fatty acids to your dog's diet (fish oils/coconut oil) can be a solve or at least a help.

SIGNS & SYMPTOMS:
- Constant licking and chewing of paws or any body part
- Skin is red with or without a foul smell
- Patches of hair may be missing

WHAT YOU MAY NEED:
- Gentle bacterial soap or oatmeal bath
- Calamine lotion
- Aloe vera gel
- Blunt-nosed scissors
- Cone collar to prevent licking/scratching
- Benadryl® (not containing Cetirizine, Acetaminophen or Pseudoephedrine) or medication prescribed by your Veterinarian

WHAT TO DO:
Cleanse the area with warm water and a mild (non-stinging) anti-bacterial soap or oatmeal shampoo. Rinsing with cooled chamomile or calendula tea may bring relief from itchiness.

Clip hair short with blunt-nosed scissors if it hinders a good examination. Using a razor may irritate the skin and hurt your dog.
Applying calamine lotion or aloe vera gel may sooth the itch but is not a long-term fix. You need to determine the source.

Try treatment for hot spots (page 191) if the area seems to be staying too moist, but truly an examination by your Veterinarian is in order to determine the cause.

1 mg Benadryl® per every pound of your dog's body weight might make him sleepy enough to stop scratching until he reaches the veterinary office, but check first to confirm that it won't

interfere with any testing that will need to be performed, medications your pet is taking or conditions your pet may have. . Also make sure Benedryl® does not contain cetirizine, acetaminophen or pseudoephedrine.

HOMEOPATHIC TIP: For allergic dermatitis and other rashes, *Rhus Toxicodenodron* may help the body alleviate symptoms. Realize that most chronic skin conditions are related to diet. Tonic herbs support your dog's system in de-toxifying allowing him to heal himself. A good basic formula is:

2 parts burdock root, 1 part dandelion, 1 part red clover and 1 part garlic powder steeped in water and cooled and fed 1 tablespoon daily per 40 lbs. of your dog's body weight. Flax, fish oil or omega-3s should also be fed daily.

STRANGLES (aka Puppy Strangles or Juvenile Cellulitis)

CONDITION OVERVIEW:
Puppy strangles is rarely seen in adult dogs and generally affects puppies under four months of age. The face, outer part of the ear (pinnae) and salivary lymph nodes are most commonly affected, and like some other diseases…we just don't know what causes it. Basically it is an immune disorder passed through the genes. A few breeds (Dachshunds, Golden Retrievers and Gordon Setters) seem more prone than others to getting strangles.

PREVENTIVE MEASURES/CAUSES:
- None available or known at this time

SIGNS/SYMPTOMS:
- Sudden and severe swelling of the face, especially eyelids, lips and muzzle; possibly enlarged salivary lymph nodes
- Pus or ooze from the facial skin or ears, skin is tender; in very rare cases, pustule nodes may be found on the trunk and other parts of the body
- Crusty lesions
- Lethargy
- Loss of appetite
- Sudden onset joint pain
- Fever

WHAT YOU MAY NEED:
- Gauze
- Chlorhexidine or mild soap for basic wound care

WHAT TO DO:
Take your puppy to the Veterinarian to determine (possibly through skin biopsy) if there could be a bacterial or infectious basis and follow prescribed treatment.

TOAD POISONING

CONDITION OVERVIEW:

Amphibians secrete a mucus through their skin to help them evade predators, but in some species this slime is toxic and can cause harm to your dog if ingested or absorbed through his skin. The Colorado River Toad (found west of the Pecos River in Southern California and the Southwestern part of the United States) and the Marine Toad (found in Hawaii and from Corpus Christi, Texas, east down the Gulf Coast into Florida) can actually kill your precious dog! The toxins can affect the heart and nervous system and lead to death.

PREVENTIVE MEASURES/CAUSES:

- Teach your dog to "leave it" and not chase after critters.
- Always be right by his side when investigating new and uncharted territory where creatures inhabit.

SIGNS & SYMPTOMS:

- Long strings of saliva coming from your pet's mouth
- Seizures
- Collapse

WHAT YOU MAY NEED:

- Water to rinse your pet's mouth
- Transportation to get your pet to help

WHAT TO DO:

Toad poisoning is a true medical emergency. Rinse your dog's mouth with water using a spray bottle for several minutes and get him to the Veterinarian keeping a watch on his vitals en route! Lean your dog's head forward or to the side, spraying so that the water drains out the mouth rather than being swallowed since you are rinsing away a toxin.

Should he demonstrate signs of shock, cardiac or pulmonary arrest, refer to those pages in this book to get you through until you reach veterinary care.

TONGUE SWELLING

CONDITION OVERVIEW:

A swollen tongue is most often a result of an allergic reaction due to bee stings, medication, food or an embedded object. Tongue swelling can be serious as it may prevent your dog from eating or even interfere with his breathing (as in the case of electrocution!) ***Medical treatment is a must***, but there are a few things you can do to reduce suffering and maybe even save your dog's life!

PREVENTIVE MEASURES/CAUSES:

- Get down on all fours to regularly observe your pet's environment from his perspective so that you can find sharp, toxic and dangerous objects before he does.

- Teach dogs to "leave it" around bees as well as electric cords. Secure wires or unplug them in rooms where pets are left alone.
- When giving new medications, be available to observe your pet for several hours after the first dose or two to make sure he doesn't have a negative reaction.

SIGNS & SYMPTOMS:
- Difficulty breathing or difficulty closing mouth
- Red and/or swollen tongue
- Drooling
- Not willing to eat or drink

WHAT YOU MAY NEED:
- Cool water
- Tweezers, gauze square or gloved fingers to remove item
- Benadryl® (not containing Cetirizine, Acetaminophen or Pseudoephedrine) if bee sting related

WHAT TO DO:
Offer cool water to your dog to alleviate discomfort and swelling.

Check for foreign object in your dog's mouth if he will let you do so without harm to yourself. Grasp his tongue with a piece of gauze and with your fingers or tweezers, remove the object. It is best to have someone else available to hold your pet while you do this.

If you suspect the swelling is due to a caustic or toxic substance, use a squirt or spray bottle with water to dilute the effects. Lean your dog's head forward or to the side, spraying so that the water drains out the mouth rather than being swallowed since you may be rinsing away a toxin.

If the swelling is due to a bee sting (see page 146) , an antihistamine might serve him best – 1mg Benedryl® per pound of your pet's body weight and monitor him closely for any additional reactions. If the swelling persists or any other symptoms such as labored breathing present themselves, get to the Veterinarian at once.

TOOTH LOSS OR DAMAGE

CONDITION OVERVIEW:
Periodontal disease (inflamed gums) is the most common reason for loss of an adult tooth in a dog. Bacteria in plaque damages the gums and connective tissue around the base of the tooth resulting in inflammation and tooth loss. A metabolic disorder known as hyperparathyroidism could also be the culprit as it reduces calcium from bones and teeth leading to tooth loss. That said, trauma (a fall or blow to the face) or chewing on hard materials (especially when getting a stick or other sharp object caught between teeth) can also result in tooth loss or damage and requires veterinary care.

PREVENTIVE MEASURES/CAUSES:
- Avoid letting your dog chew on rocks and hard items that could snap his teeth.
- Practice good dental care by brushing your pet's teeth 3-4 times weekly and getting annual veterinary exams.

SIGNS & SYMPTOMS:
- Bleeding, swelling, redness
- Drooling
- Not eating

WHAT YOU MAY NEED:
- Milk
- Cool Water
- Anbesol®
- Cotton-tipped swabs

WHAT TO DO:
Preserve any knocked-out teeth by placing them in a container of milk to protect the tissue and keep moist.

Offer your dog cool water to diminish pain and swelling and get him to the Veterinarian.

If there is a delay, your Veterinarian may suggest dabbing a small amount of Anbesol® on to a cotton swab and applying to the gum to lessen your dog's pain.

Provide soft food while your dog's mouth heals.

UNDER WEIGHT (Anorexia)

CONDITION OVERVIEW:
Some dogs are finicky eaters, but this can be a concern for any pet parent whose furry kid is considerably underweight. You should be able to feel the ribs but not see them (with some exception on Greyhounds, Rhodesian Ridgebacks and other inherently lean dogs). If ribs and hip bones are prominent, speak with your Veterinarian.

PREVENTIVE MEASURES/CAUSES:
- Problems with teeth or gums
- Stomach issues
- Sense of smell waning
- Stress/change in environment

SIGNS & SYMPTOMS:
- Not eating
- Vomiting
- Weight loss/ribs showing, eyes sunken, hair loss

WHAT YOU MAY NEED:
- Nutrient dense food prescribed by Veterinarian and supplemental vitamins

WHAT TO DO:
First, get a veterinary check-up for blood testing and to determine any underlying causes, then follow your medical professional's instructions.

If it's an older dog who may have lost their sense of smell, warming food could increase aroma and stimulate appetite.

HOMEOPATHIC TIP: If anorexia is not linked to any underlying illness, 1 30c of Alfalfa per 20 lbs. of your pet's body weight 4 times daily may increase appetite.

URINARY BLOCKAGE

CONDITION OVERVIEW:
This is a more common condition in males as the urethra (the tube draining urine from the bladder) in your female dog is wider and allows stones (inflammatory material that forms in the kidneys due to viral infections or diet) to more readily pass. When stones create a blockage, pressure increases in the upper urinary tract and the kidneys fail. Waste then builds up making the blood toxic and results in death if quick medical action is not taken.

PREVENTIVE MEASURES/CAUSES:
- Dogs should consume ½ - 1 ounce of water daily for every pound they weigh.

SIGNS & SYMPTOMS:
- Straining to urinate
- More frequent need -- dog asks to go out frequently with no output
- Inappropriate urination (in places they usually would not go) as they can't make it to the correct place in time
- Blood or dark fluid in the urine
- Distended lower abdomen, usually painful to the touch
- Later stages include loss of appetite, sluggishness and vomiting

WHAT YOU MAY NEED:
- Your observation skills -- tune in to your pet to notice his or her habits and react when they change.

WHAT TO DO:
Call your Veterinarian immediately if you notice your pet isn't releasing urine on a regular schedule. This can be excruciating to your dog and can be deadly since toxins that can't be voided end up in the blood stream and travel to the organs and tissues.

VOMITING (Emesis)

(see Diarrhea page 177)

WATER TOXICITY (Hyponatremia)

CONDITION OVERVIEW:
Hyponetremia occurs when dogs that repeatedly dive into water with their mouths open trying to catch a ball can, ingest larger quantities of water than you might suspect. Drinking too much causes electrolyte levels to drop, thins blood plasma and leads to swelling of the brain and other organs. Running/hiking dogs may tank up on too much fluids as well. This electrolyte imbalance can be fatal.

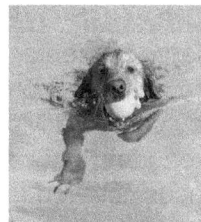

PREVENTIVE MEASURES/CAUSES:
- Give small rest breaks allowing your dog's respiration to achieve normalcy in a shady environment before consuming fluids. Also give pets a time-out from the water frequently.

SIGNS & SYMPTOMS:
- Lack of coordination
- Nausea/vomiting
- Lethargy
- Bloating
- Dilated pupils, glazed eyes
- Pale gums
- Excessive salivation

Advanced symptoms include:
- Difficulty breathing
- Collapse
- Loss of consciousness
- Seizures.

WHAT YOU MAY NEED:
- Towel or board to transport collapsed pet
- Transportation and a calm you to get professional medical help
- Electrolytes (See recipe page 174)

WHAT TO DO:
During heavy activity, provide electrolytes rather than just water.

Hyponetremia is a life-threatening emergency if in advanced stages... Get your dog to the Veterinarian or Animal ER at once!

WORMS

CONDITION OVERVIEW:
A large percentage of puppies are born with roundworms/ascarids that they received through their momma's milk. Female roundworms can produce 200,000 eggs per day so they can quickly obstruct your pet's intestines. Whipworms look like microscopic pieces of thread and are hard to diagnose due to their size but often lead to chronic weight loss and mucus covered feces. Hookworms suck blood from your dog's intestines causing anemia, bloody diarrhea and fatigue. Tapeworms get inside your dog if they ingest a flea as fleas find tapeworm eggs to be quite tasty. Tapeworms are made up of segments that when eliminated from your pet's body look like a grain of wiggling rice in his feces or around his anus.

PREVENTIVE MEASURES/CAUSES:
- Get puppies promptly de-wormed or at the first sign of worms in the feces or a bloated puppy (most need it by 4 weeks and several times until 6 months of age.)
- Apply species-specific, weight-appropriate flea treatment to keep these parasites away from your pet.

SIGNS & SYMPTOMS:
- Butt scooting
- White segments, blood or mucus in stool
- Pot-bellied appearance in puppies or kittens
- Weight-loss
- Fatigue
- Visual identification of a roundworm or tapeworm

WHAT YOU MAY NEED:
Anthelmintics are medications that expel or destroy parasitic worms without harm to the dog. Your Veterinarian needs to prescribe the type needed and proper dosage so give exactly as recommended.

WHAT TO DO:
Take a stool sample to your Veterinarian so that he or she can determine which type of worm your dog has and how to best eliminate the pesky parasite before it becomes a bigger issue.

NOTE: Heartworms are relatively easy to prevent but difficult and costly to cure, and they often result in death for our companion animals. Once again prevention is key. Get annual check-ups including blood tests as advised by your Veterinarian. Heartworm disease has been reported in all 50 states and the bite of just one mosquito infected with heartworm larvae can give your dog the disease. Use preventive medications as prescribed.
They come in monthly pills, topicals or injections and could save your dog's life!

SIGNS & SYMPTOMS:

Initially none are observed but eventually...

- Coughing
- Easily winded
- Unconsciousness from lack of blood getting to brain
- Abnormal lung sounds
- Fluid retention

NOTES:

_____

_____

_____

_____

_____

_____

_____

Dog First-Aid Conclusion

Hopefully you now feel much more confident and prepared to help any dog in your care. Knowing the skills is important, but developing the confidence to calmly and effectively react is essential to your dog's chances for recovery.

Please, please, please familiarize yourself further with this material BEFORE you need it, and practice as many of the techniques as you can. It is perfectly safe and advisable to practice muzzling and bandaging on the family dog and is important for them to become comfortable with you doing so. Just take care to cause no discomfort and never leave a muzzled pet unattended. If the first time your dog is muzzled or bandaged happens to be when he is truly injured and in pain, your task will be much more difficult and your dog's stress level will be off the charts. If he knows these tools go on and then come off from time spent practicing with you, things will go much more smoothly for you both when you actually need to accomplish the techniques. In other words…the first time you practice your skills should not be during an actual emergency!

Do not however attempt to induce vomiting, perform a choking maneuver or CPCR on a healthy animal (feel free to try on a stuffed dog though) and certainly do not give any medications if not warranted.

Read this material, practice, re-read and practice some more so that knowing what to do becomes second nature for both you and your canine patient. Then should the worst happen…you will feel confident enough to react quickly so that the two of you can safely arrive at your Veterinarian with the best possible chances for a great outcome!

It's always better to have skills and knowledge and not need them than to need them and not have them!

Paws & fingers crossed for a happy lifetime together!

There is always more to learn and it should be every pet guardian's priority to continue to learn and grow. This book serves as a strong foundation from which to build your pet care knowledge. Still, there is so much more that the authors and publisher would have loved to added to this book. All involved made it their mission to provide and prepare dog guardians for common and uncommon situations that they may encounter.

One Final Important Reminder:

Important Note Regarding Dog Care, First-Aid & CPCR Techniques Provided In This Book

If you have any questions about your dog's health, seek professional veterinary care immediately!

These instructions and the contents of this book are designed to help you keep your dog more comfortable and aid with minor problems when you are unable to get to (or are on your way to) an animal hospital.

They are not meant to be a substitute for care by a licensed veterinary professional.

No liability is assumed by the authors, publisher or any other party with respect to the information, suggestions and techniques described in this book.

Should there be any discrepancy between the suggestions offered and the advice of a Veterinarian who has knowledge of the pet in question, it is recommended that the advice of the Veterinarian be followed since the Veterinarian has the advantage of physically examining the pet and knowing its medical history and circumstances.

ABOUT THE AUTHORS

DENISE FLECK

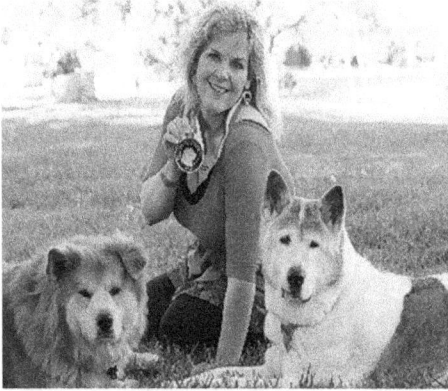

Photo by: Timothy Fielding

Denise Fleck developed the curriculum for her Pet First-Aid & CPCR Classes after training with a dozen national organizations, taking seminars to this day about everything animal, reading, practicing and serving as a long-time rescue volunteer and animal response team member. She has personally taught nearly 20,000 humans animal life-saving skills and millions more via on-air demonstrations. She assisted Homeland Security with their K9 Border Patrol First-Aid Program and developed her own line of Pet First-Aid Kits because "My students have the best of intentions but just don't get around to getting them together themselves."

Denise has shared animal life-saving skills on Animal Planet's "Groomer Has It" and "Pit Boss", A&E's "Kirstie Alley's Big Life", CBS-TV's "The Doctors", CNN Headline News, PBS-TV's "Lassie's Pet Vet" and KTLA Los Angeles as well as on radio and in magazines.

Denise has also created the curriculum for and teaches a 20-week course in Animal Care through the Burbank Unified School District's ROP Program for high school juniors & seniors at the Burbank Animal Shelter. "My proudest moment is when one student shared that he now wants to save an animal's life rather than fighting dogs like his friends. That is why I do what I do! As the proud instructor, I hope one of my students will cure a debilitating canine disease or end animal homelessness, but if each student adopts a shelter pet, shares with friends the need for spay/neuter, never harms or judges a dog by his breed alone, I'll still wag my tail."

Her other books include *Basic Bird First Aid, First Aid Basics for Rabbits & Pocket Pets, The Autumn Winter of Your Pet: Make Those Senior Years Golden, The Pet Safety Crusader's My Pet & Me Guide to Pet Disaster PAWparedness, Quickfind Books Dog First Aid & CPR, Cat First Aid & CPR, How to Take Care of Your Dog or Puppy and How to Take Care of Your Cat or Kitten; Rescue Critters Pet First Aid for Kids* and her award-winning *Don't Judge a Book by its Cover* which received the Dog Writers Association of America's Maxwell Medallion for Best Children's Book of 2014 and first sequel, *"Start off on the Right Paw"*. Denise has also won 2 MUSE Awards and 2 Special Awards from the Cat Writer's Association, 5 Maxwell Medallions from the Dog Writer's Association, Volunteer of the Year from the Burbank Police Department for her work at the Animal Shelter and has twice been a finalist as the Pet Industry's Woman of the Year.

Denise and her husband Paul live with two rescued Akitas, Haiku & Bonsai.

Learn more at www.PetSafetyCrusader.com.

ROBERT SEMROW

Robert Semrow, like so many other pet parents, was rescued by two wonderful and amazing dogs that changed his life in ways few could imagine. Sugar and Zoey were truly special beings that changed Robert's direction in life. Sugar's special needs inspired Robert to create The Pawtographer, www.thepawtographer.com.

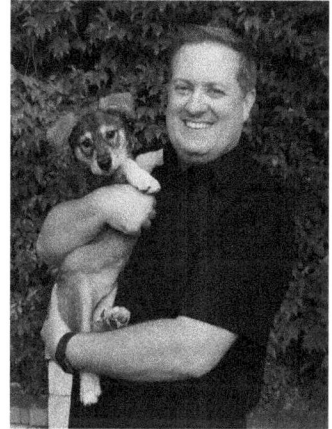

From there, Robert founded Pet World Insider, and then Pet World Media Group, a media company focused on the pet world. Robert's love and passion for the pet world led him to become deeply involved in many areas of the pet world from pet nutrition to pet safety and much more. Robert has interviewed, worked with and learned from many of the best and brightest in the pet world. His passion for the pet world is only matched by his desire to learn and share what he learns with fellow pet parents.

Robert has shared his knowledge, expertise and passion for the pet world on national television programs, via new media outlets and also on AM/FM/XM radio stations across North America. He has shared expertise on pet health, nutrition, behavior and more with audiences around the world. One of his greatest pleasures and missions is to learn and share what he learns.

Robert resides in Southern California with his wife, Amber, his daughters Amaya and Aubrey, and his beloved pets Bella Gem, Hatch and Faith.

Learn more about Robert and his projects at www.petworldinsider.com

PART III - RESOURCES

Pet Disaster PAWparedness Checklist
Pet's Health Record
Dog Head-to-Tail Chart
Poisonous Plant chart
Common Poisons List
Missing Pet Flyer
Healthy Pet Weight Chart
Body Language Visual Chart
Body Language Description Chart
Pet Vitals Chart
Pet Emergency ID Card
Pet Alert Information

PAWparedness Check List

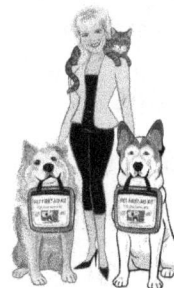

for _____

- ☐ Properly fitting Collar, Harness, Leash & Muzzle
- ☐ Crate / Carrier, Stakes / Tie-out
- ☐ Extra ID Tags
- ☐ Food (use by date _____)
- ☐ Water
- ☐ Medications / Supplements including instructions and any care / behavioral needs
- ☐ Bowls, spoon & can Opener
- ☐ Grooming Supplies (wipes, brushes, combs, clippers, etc...)
- ☐ Clean-Up Bags, Disposable Litter Pan, Litter & Scoop
- ☐ Species-specific needs
- ☐ Blankets / Bedding / Toys (shirt that smells like YOU)
- ☐ Pet Medical Records / Proof of Vaccinations
- ☐ Pictures of all pets with all family members (include identifying features)
- ☐ Disinfectant, Paper Towels, Soap
- ☐ Plastic Bags, Zip Ties, Duct Tape
- ☐ Pet First Aid Kit
- ☐ Flash Light
- ☐ Transistor Radio
- ☐ Human Supplies & First Aid Kit

www.SunnyDogInk.com

VIP Names & Numbers:

Veterinarian: _____

Animal ER: _____

Pet Sitter / Designated Caregiver #1: _____

Pet Sitter / Designated Caregiver #2: _____

Police: _____

Fire: _____

Directions To Our House & Our Phone Number:

_____

_____

MY PET'S HEALTH RECORD

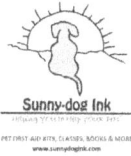

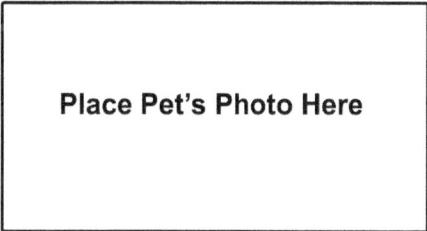

Sunny-dog Ink

PET FIRST AID KITS, CLASSES, BOOKS & MORE
www.sunnydogink.com

Date Updated: _____

Pet's Name: _____

Pet's Sex: _____   Birth Date: _____

Species: _____   Breed: _____

Weight: _____   Color(s): _____

Special Markings: _____

Normal Temperature: _____   Normal Pulse: _____   Normal Respiration: _____

Microchip #: _____   Phone Number For Microchip Agency: _____

Vaccinations: _____

_____

_____

Veterinarian: _____   Phone Number: _____

Address & Directions: _____

_____

Animal Emergency Center: _____   Phone Number: _____

Address & Directions: _____

_____

Diet: _____

Medications & Supplements: _____

_____

Daily Exercise: _____

Sleeping Location: _____

Recent Medical History: _____

_____

Place Pet's Photo Here

Average Heart Rate for Dogs and Cats

Species	Average Heart Rate
Cats	160 – 200 beats per minute
Small dogs	90 – 160 beats per minute
Medium to Large dogs	65 – 90 beats per minute

Average Respiration Rate for Dogs and Cats

Species	Average Respiration Rate
Cats and small dogs	20 – 40 breaths per minute
Medium to large dogs	10 – 30 breaths per minute

Please note: Very large dogs and/or geriatric animals may have slower respirations. Rule of thumb is the bigger and the older the dog or cat, the slower his pulse and respiration. The smaller and younger the animal, the faster their breathing and pulse.

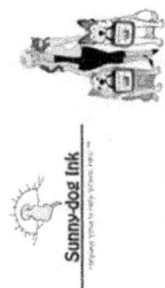

Knowing what is normal for your pet can help you determine what is not!

DOG

WEEKLY "HEAD-TO-TAIL CHECK-UP" WORKSHEETS FOR DOGS

Use this worksheet to note any bumps, lumps, irregularities, scars or surgeries your dog has.
Use a different color pen to note changes you find (size, color, smell, sensitivity etc.) and report them to your Veterinarian.

Skin
Coat / Overall appearance
Crown / Skull
Ears
Eyes / Pupils
Muzzle
Snout
Mouth
Teeth
Gums / Check capillary refill time _____
Neck
Hydration
Chest / Ribs
Abdomen
Respirations _____
Spine
Front Legs
Hind Legs
Paws (Pads, toes, claws)
Pulse _____
Tail

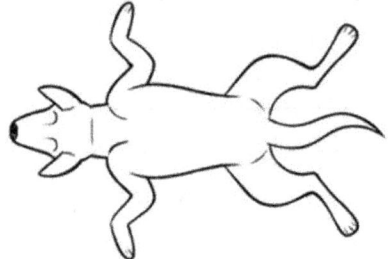

Back

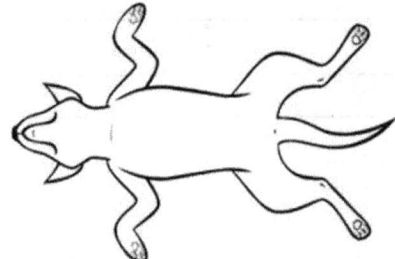

Belly

DOG'S NAME: _____
Date updated: _____

	At Rest	At Play	
Pulse	_____	_____	
Respiration	_____	_____	
Temperature	_____	_____	(Normal = 100.4° F – 102.5° F)
Capillary Refill Time	_____	_____	(2 seconds or less)
Weight	_____	_____	

Healthy Dog Weight

Work with your veterinarian to make sure pets are a healthy weight. In general, you should be able to feel and/or see a pet's ribs through a thin layer of fat. An ideal weight is an important foundation for your pet's health and well-being.

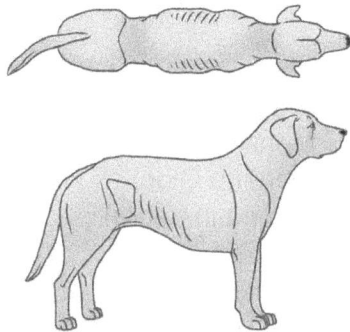

Thin to underweight, you will see or feel the ribs easily.

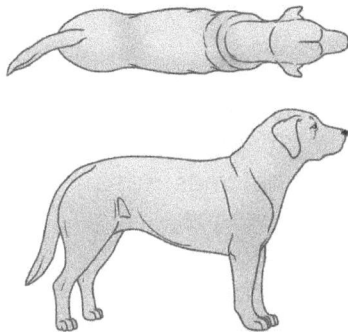

Ideal weight and a fit pet. Ribs can be felt, but not necessarily seen.

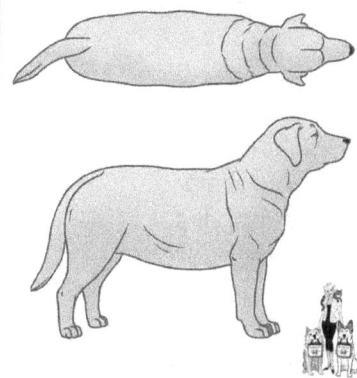

Ribs are not seen and can be difficult to feel.

Poisonous Plant List

Be diligent and always check to see if plants that your pets can interact with are safe. There are many plants that can be dangerous and have toxic effects on pets. This list is a starting point for pet parents and is not all-inclusive. This list includes some of the common plants and trees that can be poisonous or toxic to pets...

Aconite	Castor Bean	Mistletoe
African Evergreen	Chinaberry Tree	Monkshood
Alocasia	Christmas Rose	Morning Glory
Amaryllis	Cowbane	Mountain Laurel
American Holly	Daffodils	Narcissus
Angel's Trumpet	Daphne	Nightshade
Anthurium	Daylily	Oleander
Apple Tree	Dumbcane	Oriental Lily
Apricot Tree	Easter Lily	Periwinkle
Apple Leaf Croton	Elderberry	Philodendron
Arrowgrass	Elephant Ear	Pokeweed
Arrowhead Vine	English Ivy	Poinsettia
Asian Lily	Fern Palm	Poison Hemlock
Atropa Belladonna	Foxglove	Rhododendron
Autumn Crocus	Holy	Rhubarb
Azaleas	Horse Chestnut	Sago Palm
Baby's Breath	Hyacinth	Shamrock
Baneberry	Iris	Skunk Cabbage
Beech Trees	Jerusalem Cherry	Star of Bethlehem
Bird of Pradise	Jessamine	Sweet Pea
Bishops's Weed	Jimson Weed	Tiger Lily
Black Locust	Lantana	Tobacco
Bluebonnet	Larkspur	Water Hemlock
Branching Ivy	Lily of the Valley	Wisteria
Buckeye	Lupine	Yellow Oleander
Buttercup	Mayapple	Yew
Cardiac Glycosides	Milkweed	Yucca

Common Poisons List

Be diligent and observe where and what your pets can interact with. There are many hazards and dangers that are constantly present in your pets lives. Preparation, awareness and avoidance are important for the safety of your pets. The following are some of the common poisons and hazards your pet may encounter:

Household Items:

Acetaminophen Products
Antibiotics
Aspirin
Carbon Monoxide
Cigars
Coins
Deodorizers
E-Cigarettes
Fuels
Gardening Products
Kerosene
Liquid Potpurri
Medications
Pesticides
Plants
Tobacco
Windshield Wiper Fluids

Acids
Antifreeze
Batteries
Cholecalciferol
Cleaners
De-icers
Detergents
Fertilizers
Fungicides
Gardening Tools
Laxatives
Marijuana
Mothballs
Petroleum Products
Prescription Medications
Toys
Zinc

Alkaline Products
Aromatherapy Oils
Bleach
Cigarettes
Cocoa Mulch
Deodorants
Dyes
Fireworks
Herbacides
Insecticides
Lead
Matches
Paintballs
Pine Oils
Rodenticides
Tools

Foods & Consumables:

Alchohol
Caffeine
Chicken Bones
Grapes
Macadamia Nuts
Onions
Walnuts

Bones
Candy
Coffee
Gum
Mushrooms
Raisins
Xylitol Products

Bread Dough
Chocolate
Fuit Pits & Seeds
Hops
Nuts
Rhubarb Leaves

MISSING PET

Missing Since: _____

Photo of Missing Pet Here

Name: _____

Breed: _____

Color: _____

Distinguishing Features: _____

_____

_____

Female / Male: _____

Height / Length: _____

Weight: _____

Wearing ID: _____

Wearing Collar: _____

If Seen/Found Please Contact: _____

_____

_____

Special Notes:

PET ALERT

Please Rescue our
Animal Family Members:

_____Dog(s)   _____Cat(s)   _____Bird(s)
_____Other (specify)_____

Emergency Contact: _____

_____

_____

_____

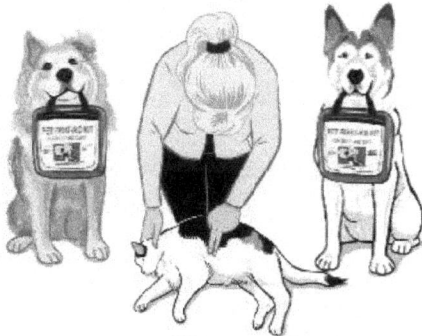

Thank you for caring!

Dog Body Language Visual Chart

It's important to be able to understand your pet's body language.
Become familiar with their audible cues and visual clues.

Happy Dog

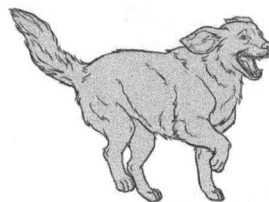

Grumpy Pup

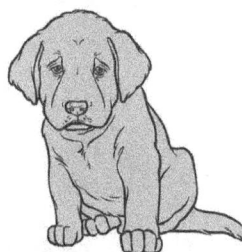

Freightened Fido

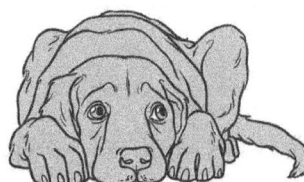

Sick Dog

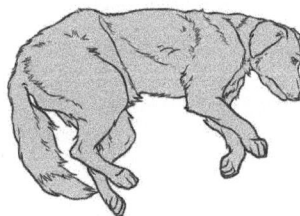

	Happy Dog	Grumpy Pup	Frightened Fido	Sick Dog
Ears	Flat	Flat & Pressed Back Against Head	Pulled Back Against Head	To The Sides Or Any Abnormal Position
Eyes	Open & Bright	Pupils Narrow	Wide Open	Half Crossed
Hackles (Fur on the neck back)	Relaxed & Smooth Fur	Fluffed Up	Fluffed Up	Could Go Either Way
Tails	Relaxed or upright especially if the tip of the tail is curled can mean "howdy" from a dog. May lower front legs with butt in the air waggin tail with a "play bow"	Swishing with hair bristled or straight up like a bottle brush; dogs may still be wagging so beware.	Tucked between legs or he'll bow with hair standing straight up.	Tucked Between Legs
Sounds	Happy bark that sounds like "Play With Me" from dogs	Low gutteral sounds or growls from dogs	Frightened cry to growing	

Your Dog's Vital Sign Record

Fill in these table so that you have a record of your dogs' vital signs.
If you only have one dog, leave the lower record for later,
when your dog enters their senior years.

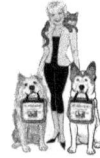

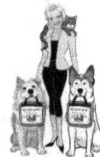

MY DOG'S VITALS

Pets Name			
	Normal	**At Rest**	**After Play**
Respiration	Medium & Large: 10-30 inhalations pet minute Small & Puppies: 20-40 inhalations per minute		
Pulse	Medium & Large: 65 - 90 beats pet minute Small & Puppies : 90 - 160 beats per minute		
Temperature	100.4°F - 102.5°F (38°C - 39.16°C)		
Weight			
Date			

Your Dog's Vital Sign Record

Fill in these table so that you have a record of your dogs' vital signs.
If you only have one dog, leave the lower record for later,
when your dog enters their senior years.

MY DOG'S VITALS

Pets Name			
	Normal	**At Rest**	**After Play**
Respiration	Medium & Large: 10-30 inhalations pet minute Small & Puppies: 20-40 inhalations per minute		
Pulse	Medium & Large: 65 - 90 beats pet minute Small & Puppies: 90 - 160 beats per minute		
Temperature	100.4°F - 102.5°F (38°C - 39.16°C)		
Weight			
Date			

Pet Emergency Identification Card

In Case of emergency please make sure my pets are cared for.

Owner Name: _____   Phone: _____

Address: _____

Alternate Contact Info: _____

I have _____ pets at home.

Urgent Medical Concerns: _____

- -

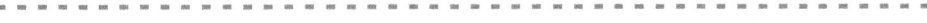

Emergency Contact Information

Name: _____   Phone: _____

Name: _____   Phone: _____

Pets At Home In Need:

Pet #1: _____

Pet #2: _____

Pet #3: _____

Pet #4: _____

Veterinarian: _____   Phone: _____

Index

A

AAFCO, 15, 17
AAHA (American Animal Hospital Association), 9, 96, 101
abdomen, 48, 83, 102, 107, 111, 116, 118, 123, 157, 208
  distended, 102, 108, 171
  lower, 118, 142
Abdominal Compression, 118
Abdominal pain, 51, 170
abnormal behaviors, 211
abnormal heart rhythms, 156
Abnormal lung sounds, 223
Abnormal swellings, 167
Abnormal temperature, 108
abrasions, 106–7, 169, 214
abscesses, 102, 129, 131, 167, 196, 206
Absorbed poisons, 204
ACE Inhibitors, 67
acetaminophen, 67, 112, 130, 146, 148, 172, 215–16, 218
acid reflux, 179
acral lick dermatitis, 191
acupressure, 27, 29
acupressure points, 29
acupuncture, 29, 93
acute infection, 57
acute moist dermatitis, 191
ACVB (American College of Veterinary Behaviorists), 63
Adaptogens, 18
Adderall, 67
Addison, 174
Adenocarcinomas, 168
ADHD Medications, 67
adhesive tape, 112, 143–44, 162–64, 181–82, 184, 207–8
Advil, 67
aerosol air fresheners, 130
aggression, 9, 59, 118, 182, 212
  late on-set, 174
Aggressive cancerous lumps, 166
aging patterns, 90, 92
aid in re-hydration, 112
airbags, 81, 87
airway, 100, 120–21, 166, 171–72
  blocked, 117
AKC (American Kennel Club), 1–2, 7
alcohol, 48–49, 67, 80, 114, 203
  containing, 193
Alcoholic beverages, 75
alcohol poisoning, 67, 78
Aleve & Motrin, 67

allergic, 130, 145–46
allergic dermatitis, 216
allergic reactions, 18, 30, 112, 117, 124, 191, 217
  severe, 145
allergies, 6, 11, 16, 18, 40, 80, 130, 148, 196, 200, 214
aloe vera, 179
Ambien, 67
American Animal Hospital Association. See AAHA
American Automobile Association (AAA), 81
American canine hepatozoonosis (ACH), 57
American College of Veterinary Behaviorists (ACVB), 63
American Food Control Officials, 15
American Heart Association, 120
American Heartworm Society, 55
American Kennel Club. See AKC
American Veterinary Society of Animal Behavior (AVSAB), 62
Anal Sac Problems, 131
anaphylaxis, 102, 146
Anaplasmosis, 57
Anbesol, 196, 219
Ancient, 2
anemia, 58, 222
  immune-mediated hemolytic, 58
anesthesia, 36, 59, 167
animal behaviorist, 9, 37, 139
Animal Communication, 9, 29
Animal Emergency Center, 10, 75
animal hospital, 125, 147, 225
animal massage therapist, 20
Animal Poison Control Center, 74, 112, 204
annual check-ups, 9, 42, 159–60, 176, 200, 222
anorexia, 219–20
antacid, 136, 178
Antacid-coated aspirin, 112, 197
Anthelmintics, 222
Antibacterial cream, 141
antibacterial properties, 193
antibacterial soap, 61, 131, 141, 153–54, 197–98, 207
antibiotics, 53, 149, 154, 162–63, 186, 207
  oral, 193
  prescribe, 129
antibodies, 18, 29, 49–50, 154
anti-convulsants, 34
Antidepressants, 67
antidote, 75, 154
antifreeze, 73
anti-fungal treatment, 56
antigens, 50
  injected, 49
antihistamine, 112, 146, 148, 195, 218
antioxidants, 18, 74, 201, 210
antivenin, 10, 71, 101, 149, 154
ants, 69, 146
anus, 48, 132, 222
anxiety, 30, 34, 82, 84, 202, 212
Apis Meliffica, 127, 147

blood sample, 49
blood seeps, 152
blood spurts, 140
bloodstream, 46, 52, 55, 73, 120, 129, 146-47, 159, 168, 220
  pet's, 75
blood sugar, 159, 176
  high, 160–61
  low, 120, 159–60, 211
  normal, 159
blood supply, 31, 107, 206
blood tests, 129, 159, 200, 222
blood vessels, 74, 114, 140, 144, 146, 152, 185, 199
blood work, 133
bloody diarrhea, 222
  severe, 52
blunt-nosed scissors, 112, 129, 131, 138, 141, 162, 164, 192, 215
body heat, 72, 112, 160, 185, 214
body itching, 50
body language, 35, 37, 128
  changing, 97
Body Language Description Chart Pet Vitals Chart, 229
body odor, 130
body temperature, 65, 97–98, 163, 185, 189–90, 202, 213
body weight, 74, 83, 106, 121, 174–75, 179, 201, 203, 214–16
bone meal, 15, 71
bone protrusion, 197
bones, 15, 28, 30, 41, 57, 77–78, 80, 93, 106, 116–17, 168, 197–98, 218
  broken, 90, 169, 183, 197
  cooked, 170
  fragile, 27
  hip, 21, 219
  inflicting, 206
  large, 117
booster shots, 49
Bordetella, 50, 64
Bordetella bronchiseptica, 53
Brachial, 129
Brachial Artery, 142
brachycephalic, 2, 110, 137, 189, 203
brain, 19, 31, 91, 120, 123, 144, 187, 211–12, 214, 221, 223
brain cells, 97, 173, 180
brain damage, 82, 97–98, 124, 189
  permanent, 70, 72
brain tumor, 211
breathe, 97, 116, 122, 124, 143, 184, 210
breathing, 96–97, 99–100, 119–20, 122, 124, 126, 160, 166, 169, 180–81, 183–84, 186, 201–2, 204, 208–10
  labored, 218

shallow, 117
  stopped, 98, 100
breathing capacity, 20
breathing difficulties, 2, 69, 108, 111, 145, 147–48, 162–63, 171
breaths, 6, 28, 104, 109, 120, 122–23, 125, 153, 166, 184, 208
  artificial, 125
broccoli, 80, 201
Brown Recluse, 148–49
bruising, 58, 151, 167, 198
bumps, 11, 38, 42–43, 76, 106–7, 196
Bumps & Lumps, 166
burned areas, 163–64
burned paws, 68, 90
burn paws, 70, 161, 189
burns, 48, 72, 77–78, 89, 112, 161, 163–66, 169, 193, 203
Butt scooting, 131, 222

C

Caesarean, 58
cage dryers, 189
cages, 82, 85
  damaged, 89
  wire, 8, 81
calamine lotion, 215
calcium, 16, 137, 218
Can-a-bid-i-ol, 33, 133
cancer, 7, 18, 49, 166–68, 199
  uterine, 59
canine distemper, 51
Canine Erlichiosis, 199
Canine Flu, 53
Canine Heimlich, 98
canine influenza, 53
canine nutrition, 18, 200
Canine nutritionists, 157, 201, 215
canine pancreatitis, 68
canine patient, 97, 142, 148, 161, 224
Canine Sarcoptic, 195
cannabinoids, 33, 133–34
cannabis sativa, 33, 134
  plant genus, 33, 133
Canned Pumpkin Puree, 170
Capillary Bleeding, 140
capillary refill, 202
capillary refill time, 42, 105, 145, 209, 213
Capillary Refill Time. See CRT
Carbon Monoxide Poisoning, 31, 204, 210
CARDIAC PUMP METHOD, 121
cardiac stimulant, 201
Cardio Pulmonary Cerebral Resuscitation. See CPCR
Cardio Pulmonary Resuscitation. See CPR
cardiovascular disease, 7
Carprofen, 133

Distemper, 50, 55, 64, 211
Distended lower abdomen, 220
drinking habits, 174
drinking supply, 90
Drooling, 117, 147, 149, 153, 168, 202, 218–19
  excessive, 46, 196
drowning, 68, 71, 120, 124, 179
Dry hacking cough, 53
dry heaves, 158
Dystocia, 137

E

ear canals, 47, 106, 115, 173, 188
ear drum, 106, 173
ear flaps, 188, 191
ear infections, 40, 189
  inner, 136
Ear Injuries, 144
ear mites, 188
ears, 39, 41, 43, 46–47, 80, 83, 106, 109–10, 136, 140, 144, 173, 183–84, 188–90, 216
  cleaning, 188
  clipping, 188
  downward, 144
  floppy, 141, 191
  inner, 52, 136, 173, 188
  non-hearing, 173
  upright, 144, 150
  warm, 185
earthquake, 89–90, 183
ear tips, 150, 161
ear wash, 106, 188
eating, 5, 41, 53, 55–56, 80, 107, 156, 171, 176–77, 196, 217, 219
eating feces, 55
Eclampsia, 137
E-Collar, 129–30
ECS. See Endocannabinoid System
effleurage, 26–28
elastic recoil, 121
elbows, 20, 103, 115, 118, 121
  lock, 121
Electrical Burns, 165
Electric outlets, 67
electrocution, 120, 165–66, 213, 217
electrolyte imbalances, 52, 221
electrolyte replenisher, 178
electrolytes, 105, 178, 214, 221
Electrostimulation, 29
Embedded Objects, 117, 181, 217
Emergency Situations, 59, 81, 86, 98, 100, 145
emergency surgery, 156, 158
emergency veterinary care, 197
emergency veterinary hospital, 154
Emesis, 203, 220

Endocannabinoid System (ECS), 33–34, 134
Endocrine diseases, 174
endorphins, 7, 29–30
Enlarged colon, 170
Enlarged Liver, 160
Enlarged Lymph Nodes, 58
epilepsy, 33, 211
epileptic animal, 102
epi-pen, 146
Epsom Salt Solution, 129
equilibrium, 136
Erhlichia, 57
Esbilac, 61–62
esophagus, 15, 23, 78, 116, 177
Essential Fatty Acids, 93
essential oils work, 30
Estim, 29
Estradiol, 67
estrogen, 67, 139
estrogen levels, 193
estrus, 193–94
exams, 106, 188
  senior wellness, 90
Excessive panting, 108
Excessive salivation, 221
exercise, 11, 19–21, 25, 27, 30, 40, 42–43, 72, 76, 84–85, 91–92, 167, 171, 174, 200
extremities, 184
  cold, 213
eyeballs, 77, 205
eye color, 60
eye dropper, 61, 75, 112, 136, 138, 146, 160, 175, 179, 190, 202
eye injuries, 37, 109, 182
eyelid, 105, 140, 182, 195, 205, 216
eye movement, 106, 136
eyes sunken, 219
eye wash, 106, 112, 141, 182–83, 204
  sterile, 183

F

facial expressions, 106
facilities, 10, 87, 89
fallopian tubes, 59
fangs, 148–49, 151
fats, 17, 59, 75, 105, 177, 200, 204
  cook, 80
  cooked, 80
  metabolize, 80
fatty acids, adding, 215
Fatty acid supplements, 195
Fatty table scraps, 67
FDA standards, 17
Fear Free, 9, 101
feces, 52, 55, 60, 63, 222

P

Pacing, 187
pads, 65, 70, 73, 107, 134, 143, 190
  foot, 189
  gauze encircling, 143
  heating, 65, 185
  non-stick, 163–64
  secure flat, 143
pain, 20, 25–26, 34, 90–92, 95, 97–99, 102–3, 109, 132–34, 147–49, 168–70, 184, 196–98, 205–7, 219
  extreme, 182, 198
  great, 155, 162
  joint, 57, 216
  localized, 147, 149
  muscle, 52, 57
  severe, 163
  stinging, 147
pain levels, 30, 198
pain medications, 148–49, 154
palate, soft, 209
pale, 58, 105, 117, 145, 158, 185, 213
pale stool, 51
pale tongue, 51
pancreas, 77, 159
pancreatitis, 75, 77, 80, 176, 179
panting, 69, 104, 189, 196, 213
  heavy, 190, 199, 202
  started, 96
papain, 146
Parainfluenza, 50
paralysis, 148–49, 152–53, 183
  facial, 188
  temporary, 78
paraphimosis, 205–6
parasite preventives, 21
  monthly, 214
parasites, 43, 48, 54–55, 57, 68, 71, 106–7, 187, 205, 214, 222
  gastrointestinal, 205
  harbors, 107
  intestinal, 55
  pesky, 222
Parinfluenza, 64
Parvo, 52
  contract, 52
Parvovirus, 50, 52, 63–64
Patella Luxation, 132
pawing, 117, 145, 171, 182, 188, 196, 202
paw pads, 43, 143
paws, 38, 62, 66, 69–70, 72, 85, 143, 177, 181–82, 184–86, 190–92, 200, 204, 210, 215
  frozen, 185
  injured, 143
  wipe, 73
PCR Hemp Oil, 34

Pedialyte, 112, 178
pee stream, 66
pellets, 147
  slug bait, 211
  small, 127
penis, 205–6
Pepcid, 178
Pepto-Bismol, 178
perforations, intestinal, 79
Periodontal disease, 218
peroxide, 49
  hydrogen, 75, 112, 202–3
pest control methods, 34
pesticides, 5, 42
Pet Alert Information, 229
Pet Alert Sticker, 87
Pet Disaster Pawparedness Checklist, 88
Pet Disaster PAWparedness Checklist Pet's Health Record, 229
Pet Emergency ID Card, 229
Pet First-Aid & CPCR, 2, 64, 83, 96, 97, 119
Pet First-Aid Class, 64, 119, 226
Pet First-Aid Kits, 8, 193, 226
Pet First-Aid technique, 96
pet food industry, 14
pet food labels, 14, 16, 200
pet food manufacturers, 17
petit mal classifications, 211
pet nutritionist, 18, 42
Pet Obesity Prevention, 200
pet overpopulation, 58
Pet Poison Helpline, 67, 70, 201–2
pet ramp, 179
pet restraint, 82
petrissage, 26, 28
Petroleum, 186
petroleum jelly, 48, 104, 150, 186
pet-safe preventives, 68
pet safety, 65, 227
Pet Safety Crusader, 226
Pet Safety Page, 98
pet savvy, 40, 78
pet's body, 13, 18, 20, 28, 42–43, 46, 69, 113, 135, 164, 174, 182, 203, 222
pet's body weight, 69, 130, 155, 172, 195, 218, 220
pet's caregiver, 11–12
pet's chest, 107
pet scoots, 131
pets coughing, 171
pet's ears, 106, 150, 173
pet seatbelt, special, 81
Pet's Health & Safety Team, 101
Pet's Health Record, 12
Pet Sitters International, 11
pet stores, 8, 81
Pet Stretcher, 134
petting, 22, 37, 40, 168

V

Vaccinate, 49–52, 54–55
vaccinations, 9, 21, 49–50, 53, 63–64, 73, 82, 88, 154, 207
  annual, 166
  frequent, 54
  multiple, 52
  regular, 49
vaccines, 49, 52–54, 177

Valentine's Day, 74
vegetables, 16, 70
  adding raw, 18
venom, 127, 147, 149, 151–52, 154
  amount of, 147, 152
  potent, 152
ventilation, 77, 84
ventricles, 121
  right, 121
vertebrae, 28, 134
  displaced, 30
  restoring misaligned, 30
Vestibular system, 136
vet, 27, 42, 49, 54, 73, 86, 91, 137, 167, 193, 195–96
Veterinarian, 9–11, 48–50, 90–93, 101–2, 106–7, 112–15, 126–34, 136–39, 146–47, 157–64, 166–67, 169–73, 187–88, 198–207, 212–22
veterinary, 16, 114, 124, 126, 130, 139, 144, 147, 171, 173, 179–80, 182, 210, 212, 220
  annual, 13, 166
  licensed, 225
  pre-travel, 84
Veterinary Emergency & Critical Care, 121
Veterinary Orthopedic Manipulation, 30
vials, 113, 154
vinegar, white, 71, 146, 155
viral infections, 220
virus, 50, 52, 54
viruses, 50, 53
  flu, 53
vitals, 103, 105, 145, 185, 202, 209, 213, 217
vitamin deficiencies, 15
vitamin injection, 185
vitamins, 16, 18, 93, 112, 210
vomit, 55, 109, 117, 137, 158, 175, 179, 203–4
vomiting, 50–52, 57, 60, 72, 74–75, 79, 108, 111–12, 148–49, 170, 174, 176–79, 201–4, 219–21, 224
  inducing, 98, 202
  prolonged, 203
Vomiting & Diarrhea, 145

W

Warm Compress, 129
Wasps, 146
water, 16–17, 60–61, 69–72, 84–90, 105, 146, 159, 163–65, 169, 174–75, 177–80, 190–91, 204–5, 216–18, 220–21
  chemical, 179
  cold, 180
  contaminated, 55, 90
  distilled, 127
  double, 36
  drink, 68, 79, 209
  hot, 61, 193
  ice, 147, 162, 196
  luke-warm, 190
  outdoor, 189
  purified, 106, 141, 181–82, 196, 204
  room temperature, 162–64
  salt, 155
  standing, 67, 90
  tap, 69, 90
water consumption, 170
Water Toxicity, 179, 221
watery eyes, 6
Weakened muscle tone, 139
weakness, 57, 160, 168
weaning period, 62
weight, 16–17, 19, 34, 56, 60, 85, 87, 91, 202, 219
  excess, 91
  healthy, 133, 176
  losing, 107, 138
  pet's, 178
  total, 17
weight-appropriate flea treatment, 222
Weight loss, 46, 51, 54, 56–58, 160, 167, 178, 219
Weight-loss, 222
Well-oxygenated blood flow, 91
well-ventilated area, 189
wheel-barrow method, 118
wheezing, 60, 115, 199
whining, 37, 211
Whipworms, 222
White chocolate, 74
wildfires, 89
window screens, 147
windpipe, 98, 116, 171, 177, 180
winter hazards, 69
wires, 77, 165
  electrical, 165
witch hazel, 190
Wood's Lamp, 56
worms, 56, 205, 222
wound care, basic, 216
wound re-start, 144

wounds, 96, 98, 108, 110, 112, 141, 143–44,
149–50, 162, 165, 191, 193, 197, 199, 207–8
  contaminate, 162
  large, 144
  lick, 141
  minor, 112
  open, 129, 193
  sucking, 207–8
  surrounding, 129
wound site, 112
wound treatment, 166

X

Xanax, 67
x-rays, 10, 30, 137, 187, 206
xylitol, 67, 112, 159, 203, 211
  containing, 159
xylitol gum, 203

Y

Yellow Sac, 148
yogurt, 17
  non-fat, 202, 204

Z

Zestril, 67
Zocor, 67
Zooeyia, 6, 40
Zoonoses, 6, 55
Zoonotic Diseases, 51, 54–55

www.ingramcontent.com/pod-product-compliance
Lightning Source LLC
Chambersburg PA
CBHW081155020426
42333CB00020B/2506